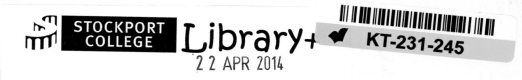
Darcey Bussell
PILATES FOR LIFE
A practical introduction to the core programme

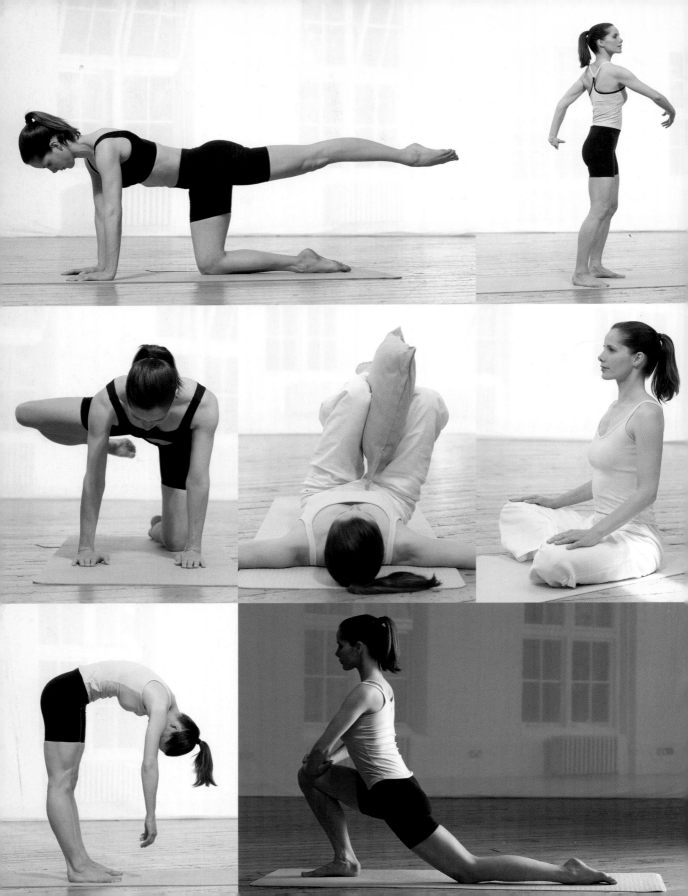

Darcey Bussell

PILATES FOR LIFE

A practical introduction to the core programme

MICHAEL JOSEPH
an imprint of
PENGUIN BOOKS

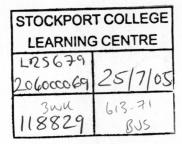
MICHAEL JOSEPH

Published by the Penguin Group
Penguin Books Ltd, 80 Strand, London WC2R 0RL, England
Penguin Group (USA) Inc., 375 Hudson Street, New York, New York 10014, USA
Penguin Books Australia Ltd, 250 Camberwell Road, Camberwell, Victoria 3124, Australia
Penguin Books Canada Ltd, 10 Alcorn Avenue, Toronto, Ontario, Canada M4V 3B2
Penguin Books India (P) Ltd, 11 Community Centre, Panchsheel Park, New Delhi - 110 017, India
Penguin Group (NZ), cnr Airborne and Rosedale Roads, Albany, Auckland 1310, New Zealand
Penguin Books (South Africa) (Pty) Ltd, 24 Sturdee Avenue, Rosebank 2196, South Africa

Penguin Books Ltd, Registered Offices: 80 Strand, London WC2R 0RL, England

www.penguin.com

First published 2005
2

All photographs by Iain Philpott, except for pages 182–3, 188, 189, 192. Copyright © Bill Cooper, 2005

Special thanks to Marks & Spencer/View From for providing Darcey's outfits

The moral right of the author has been asserted

Set in Parisine Clair
Designed by Ash
Colour Reproduction by Dot Gradations Ltd, UK
Printed in Italy by Graphicom srl

A CIP catalogue record for this book is available from the British Library

ISBN 0-718-14766-9

If you have a medical condition, are pregnant or suffer from
back problems, the exercises described in this book should not
be followed without first consulting your doctor or seeking expert
advice. All guidelines and warnings should be read carefully and
the author and publishers cannot accept responsibility for injuries
or damage arising out of a failure to do so.

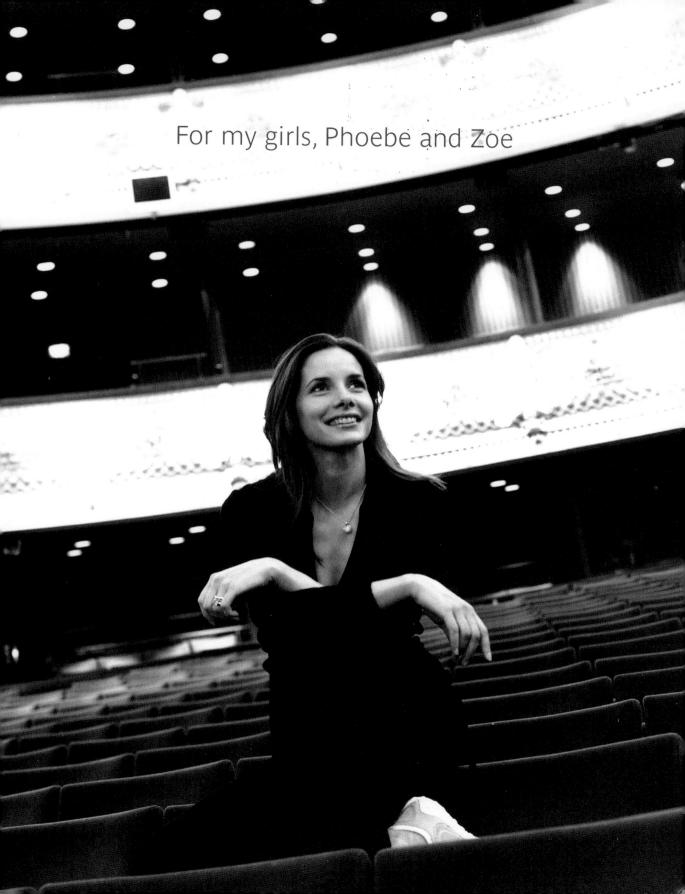

For my girls, Phoebe and Zoe

Contents

'In ten sessions you will feel the difference, in twenty you will see the difference, and in thirty you will have a whole new body'

JOSEPH H. PILATES

Introduction

I put this book together because I really believe in Pilates and how it can enhance your life. I came across the technique by chance when I was sixteen years old and, while I am not a Pilates teacher, I have been doing it enthusiastically for the whole of my professional life. I feel Pilates is the best thing I have ever done for my body, and, once you work through the exercises, I'm sure you will feel the same way too – especially if like most women you're looking for a flat stomach, taut bottom, toned arms and firm thighs. Or if you're a man looking to build core strength and lengthen your muscles, Pilates can definitely help you to achieve all this. Plus, as I have found, it's a wonderful source of meditation and relaxation. It's a form of exercise I love and I hope you will too.

Pilates (pronounced Pil-ah-tes) is basically a method of body conditioning that was developed nearly a hundred years ago in Germany by Joseph H. Pilates. It's unique because, unlike others forms of exercise, the technique works on strengthening, lengthening and toning muscles, as well as improving posture and

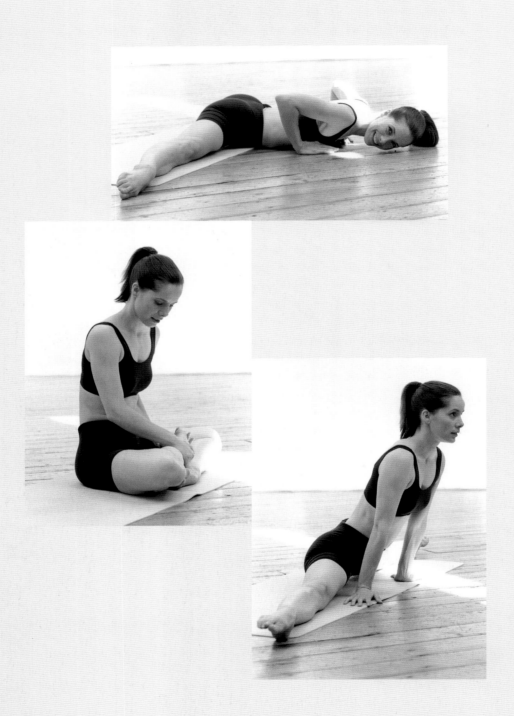

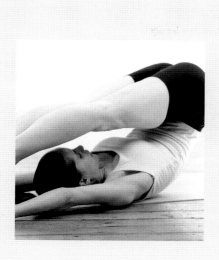

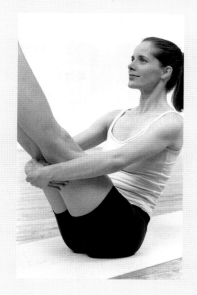

increasing your flexibility and balance. This leads to a leaner, stronger and more streamlined physique. Joseph Pilates first developed the technique to help strengthen his frail body after being plagued with asthma and rickets as a child. Interned during the First World War, he taught his method to fellow internees and successfully helped keep them strong and healthy until the war ended.

Moving to America in 1926 he set up his first Pilates studio in New York, where the Pilates method quickly became popular among dancers when Martha Graham and George Balanchine became fans. Today, Pilates is famous worldwide thanks to a devout following of dancers and celebrities, but it's also loved and adored by anyone who is looking to change their shape and achieve a strong, lithe body.

I was introduced to Pilates because as a young dancer I was very supple and needed to know how to control my body. Pilates was an excellent way for me to learn how to do this. On the whole dancers use this method because it is the best

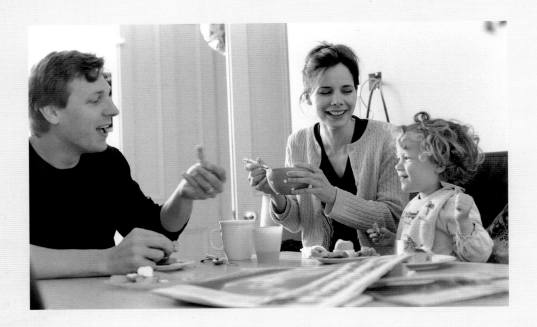

way to exercise every muscle in the body without over-developing anything and creating bulk muscle. This is especially important for us, because we don't want to appear muscle-bound on stage. In addition, the lengthening and strengthening basis of the method helps keep our muscles supple, which means we look leaner and stay stronger as dancers for longer.

Pilates is also invaluable because a lot of dancers have injuries, particularly now ballet has become so intensively athletic and our bodies inevitably pay the price in some way. Pilates has long been known as an excellent recovery tool because it can help pinpoint an injured area, isolate the muscle group that's damaged and focus specific exercises on it. Unfortunately I have had to have two ankle operations, one of which kept me from performing for nine months. Having Pilates to keep me strong through my rehabilitation helped me stay in mental and physical shape and eventually recover completely from such a serious injury.

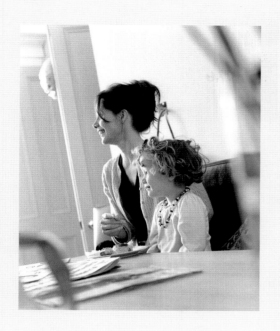

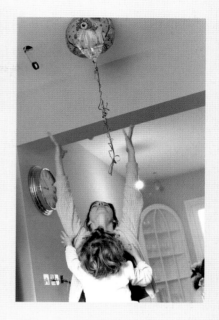

If you think Pilates looks and sounds daunting, don't worry, you don't have to be a ballet dancer to do it, and Pilates can be done by anyone of any age. The core Pilates programme I have put together in this book is for those looking to change their physique, streamline their body and improve on their posture. For beginners, I suggest doing it three times a week for an hour. When working your way through this programme you may find you get frustrated because the exercises are slow and you won't feel the burn and sweat like you do at the gym, but stick with it because as you advance you will not only feel your muscles toning up but also see your body tightening. If you have any injuries, seek medical advice before you start the programme and make sure you stop doing any exercise that gives you a sharp pain (a dull pain is your body stretching). However, whether you're in good shape or not, always work at a slow and controlled pace so you can get to grips with the exercises.

The real beauty of Pilates is that once you have mastered the exercises you can

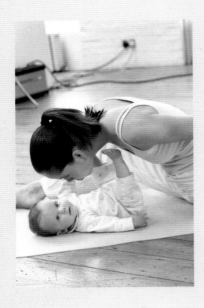

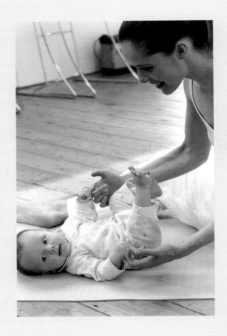

use the technique in all areas of your life because they not only make you stronger, but also teach you to become aware of your body and how you use it. Pilates shows you how to breathe and relax properly, which is essential for anyone who feels stressed out by their daily life. I do an hour and a half class twice a week, and I find that stops me being excessive about exercise, and at the same time does enough for my body.

I really feel incredibly lucky that I am able to have a career that I love and a family I adore, and I believe it's important not to get set in your ways and always stay open to new things. If you feel the same way about life, Pilates is for you because it will help you see that you can change your body and strengthen your mind no matter what your age, or what you've done in your life so far. Pilates gives me ultimate confidence. If I've done my exercises before I start my working day, I know I am prepared and ready for anything that comes my way.

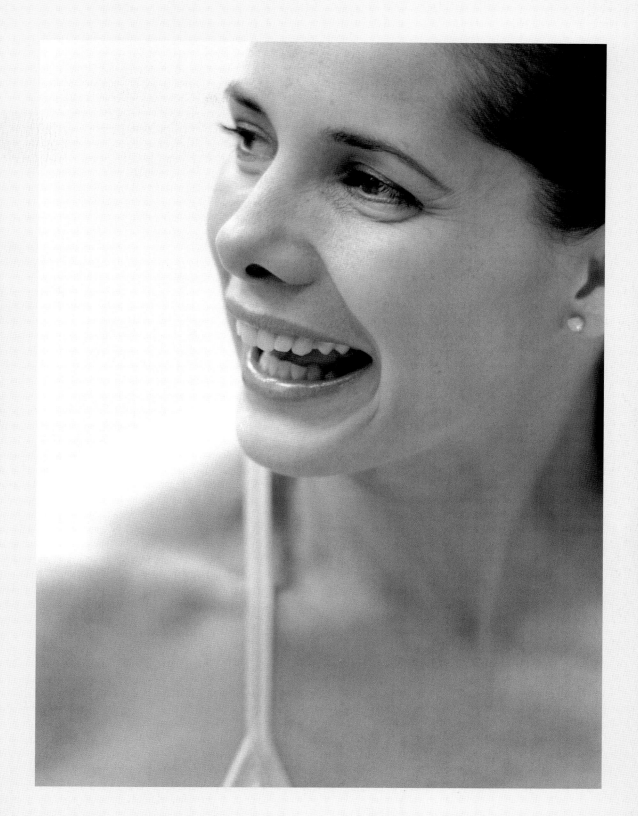

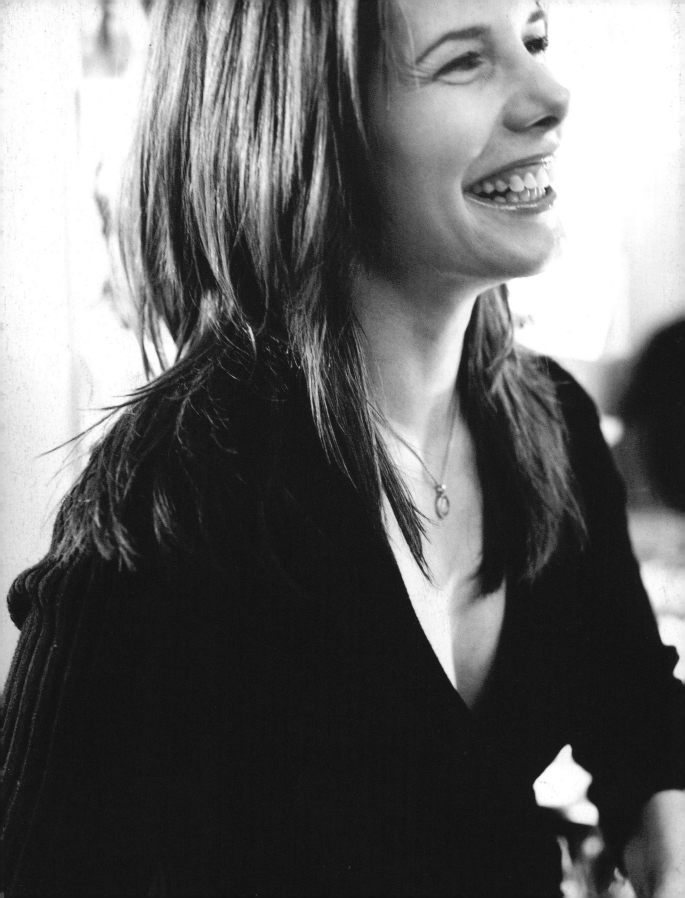

PILATES BASICS —
KEY STARTER POINTS

To gain the most from this Pilates programme it is important to understand the key elements of the Pilates technique, which are crucial to engage while doing the exercises. The following seven exercises will help you find these elements before you start. They can be done daily not only as a warm up to the core programme, but also as an excellent way to help the Pilates technique become second nature to you.

core/centre

Your core or centre is the band of muscles which wrap around your body like a corset, helping support you and giving you good posture. It is a crucial element of Pilates because every exercise requires you to initiate all movement from your core. To find your core simply pull your belly button back towards your spine.

To find your core muscles, a good cheat's exercise is to lie flat on the floor and try to push your spine onto the ground by pulling your belly button towards it. Be careful not to pull in so far that you can't breathe and your ribs stick out. The aim is to activate your abdominal muscles so your stomach goes flat, but you can still breathe normally.

Repeat ten times.

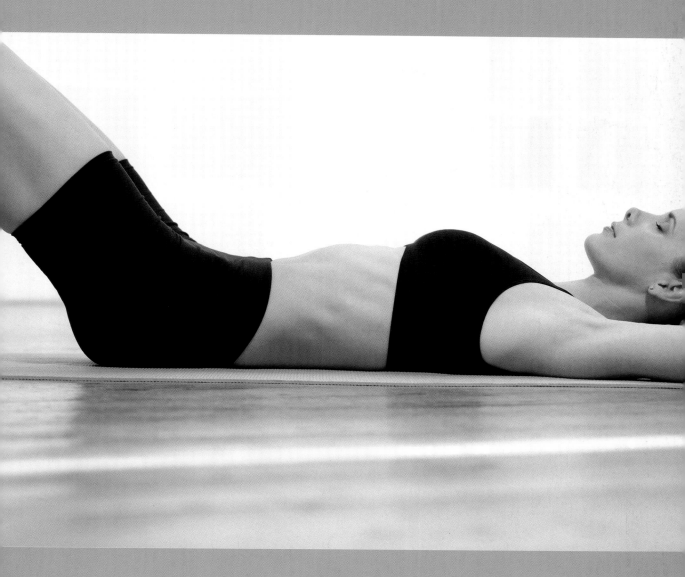

A neutral spine is the ideal position for your back during floor exercises as it places the least amount of stress on your spine. Contrary to popular belief, your spine should never be flat on the floor when lying down; there should always be a natural curve to your lower back.

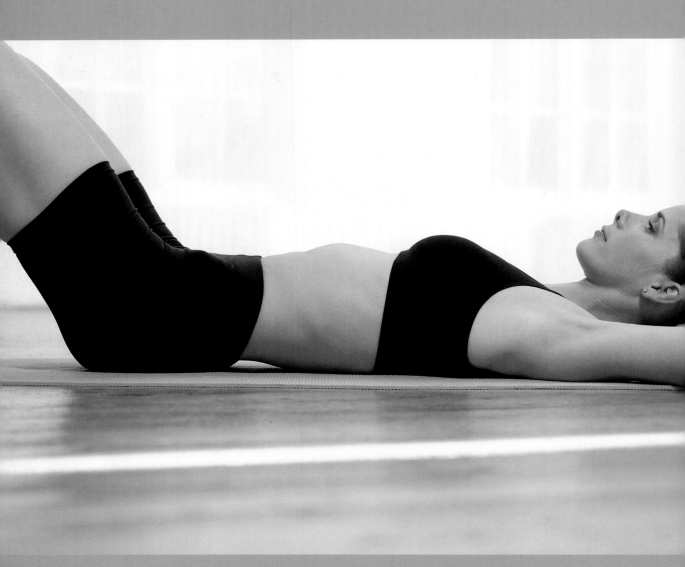

neutral spine

1   To find the correct position, lie on the floor on your back with your knees bent at a ninety-degree angle, feet in parallel and hip-width apart.

2   In this position there should be a small curve to your lower back; this means your back shouldn't be either pressed/pushed into the floor, or arched so there is a large gap between you and the floor.

3   When you are in neutral your tailbone should be dropped into the floor and there should be a small gap between your waist and the floor (ideally this should be half a flat hand).

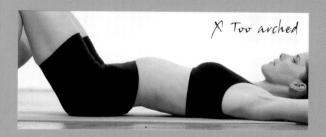

X Too arched

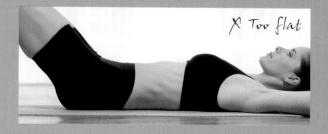

X Too flat

pelvic floor muscles

1 Lie down on the floor on your back with your legs straight and hip-width apart. Place your arms by your sides. Now, imagine peeing and then stopping mid flow – the muscles you are using are your pelvic floor muscles.

2 Squeeze these muscles together. This should allow you to feel your pelvic floor pull upwards to your stomach. Hold it for four counts, then relax.

Repeat ten times.

The pelvic floor muscles are essential to core stability as they connect to the abdominal muscles; this means your pelvic floor muscles should always be engaged when your abdominals are. If your pelvic floor loses tone, your posture will collapse and this can lead to back pain.

TIP

IF YOU'RE FINDING IT DIFFICULT TO LOCATE YOUR PELVIC FLOOR MUSCLES LIKE THIS, ANOTHER WAY TO FIND THEM IS TO SQUEEZE YOUR BOTTOM CHEEKS TOGETHER – BUT MAKE SURE YOU KEEP YOUR SPINE IN NEUTRAL WHEN YOU DO THIS.

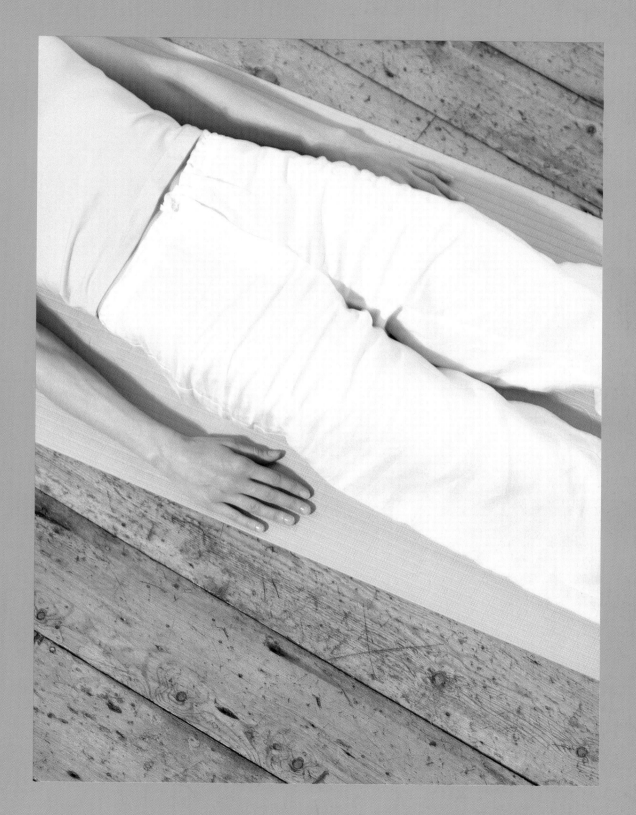

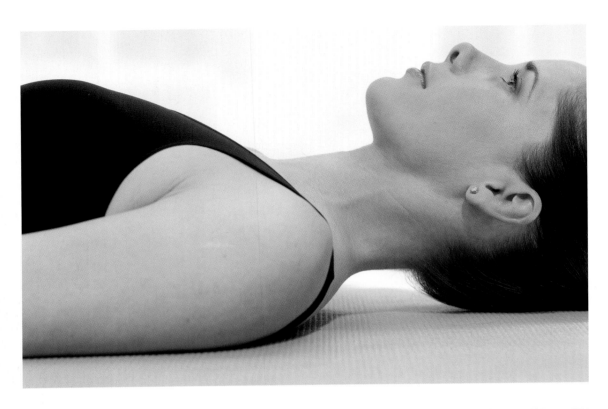

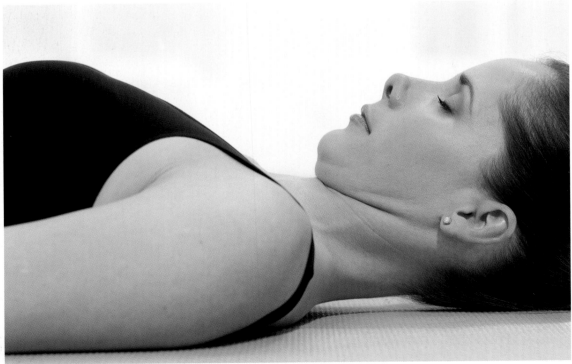

lengthening of the neck

1 Lie down on the floor on your back with your knees bent at a ninety-degree angle, feet in parallel and hip-width apart.

2 Drop your chin to your chest and inhale. As you exhale, imagine your neck lengthening away from your spine (don't force the movement).

3 For an extra neck stretch, stay in this position and do small figures of eight leading with your nose.

Repeat the circles five times in one direction and then five in the other.

The correct neck position is also essential in Pilates to help avoid injury. Whether you're lying, standing or sitting always imagine your chin moving back closer to your neck and the crown of your head being pulled upwards by a string (if you do this correctly your body will automatically move into a strong postural position).

shoulder stabilization

Many people suffer from sore shoulders and neck pain simply because they don't hold their shoulder blades stable when they raise their arms. This means for most of the day the shoulders are lifted and held in a position rather than kept in a relaxed state. In Pilates, exercises with the arms always begin with the shoulder blades sliding down the back so that the shoulders are stabilized.

1   To find this position, stand in front of a mirror with your arms by your sides. Before you start, slide your shoulder blades down your back.

2   Now, raise one arm up above your head, keeping your shoulders down. There should be no tension in the shoulder and ample space between your ear and shoulder.

Repeat with the other arm.

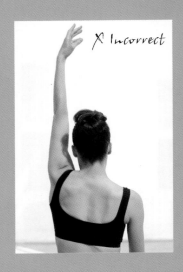

X Incorrect

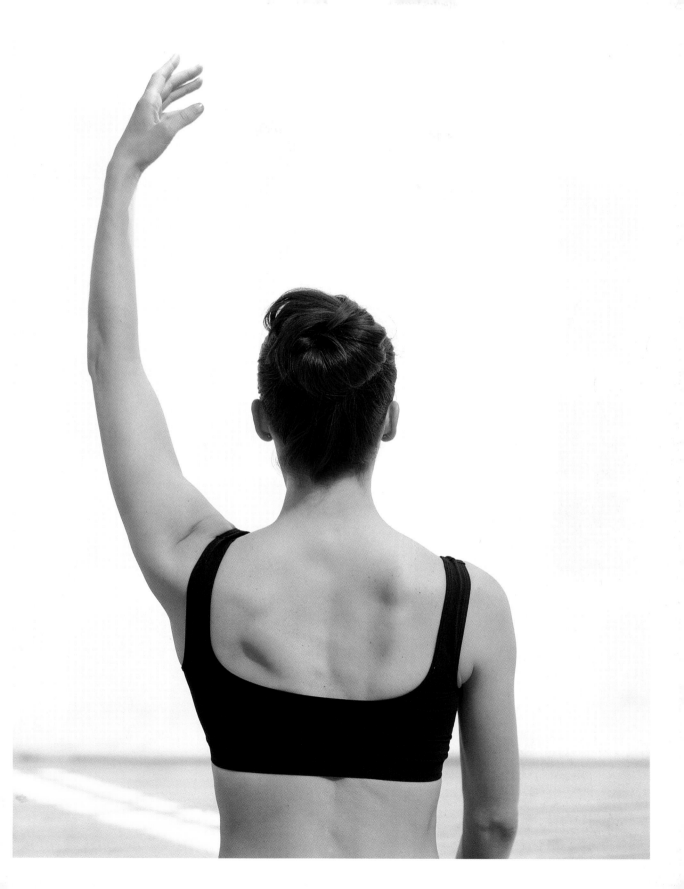

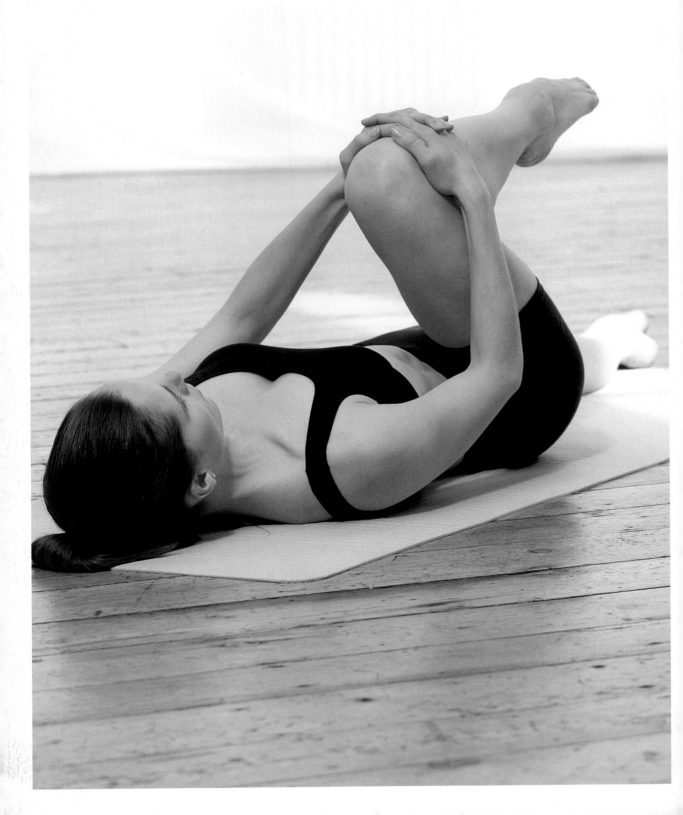

rotation of the leg or turn out

When you ask someone to turn out their leg people often think the movement comes from their feet, when in fact a leg rotation starts from the hip joint. To find the turn out, lie on the floor and put your hands on the top of your hips. Turn your legs out, focussing your attention on the tops of your thighs, rotating them outwards, down and around to the floor. In the right position the inner-thigh muscles will also engage.

1   Lie on the floor with your legs out in front of you. Now, bend one leg and lift your foot off the floor, bringing your knee up towards your chest (keep your other leg straight). Holding this knee with both hands rotate the knee by making a circle in the air with it.

2   Only the hip of the moving leg should move; the other should remain on the floor. Hold this hip down with one hand if it does move.

Do ten hip circles on each side.

the mind–body connection

Like yoga and other holistic forms of exercise Pilates has a strong mind–body connection. If you focus your mind on individual muscles as you work through the programme you can help lengthen and strengthen them. It's important to be aware all the time of how you're holding and moving your body so you can help your muscles work through their full range of movement.

1   Stand straight with your feet parallel and hip-width apart, your belly button pulled into your spine, your ribs dropped (imagine them sliding down your front), your shoulders relaxed and your head in alignment with your spine.

2   Inhale and drop your head to your chest. Exhaling, allow your arms to fall forwards as you roll down vertebra by vertebra, concentrating on each one as you move. Keep your legs straight and make sure you don't rock forwards or backwards as you move. Let go of your head and allow your hands to come as close to the floor as possible without straining.

3   Inhale at the bottom and hold the position for two counts, then exhale and, using your stomach muscles, curl upwards to return to the starting position.

Repeat three times.

> TIP
>
> IF YOU FEEL AS THOUGH YOU'RE FORCING THE MOVEMENT KEEP YOUR KNEES SLIGHTLY BENT.

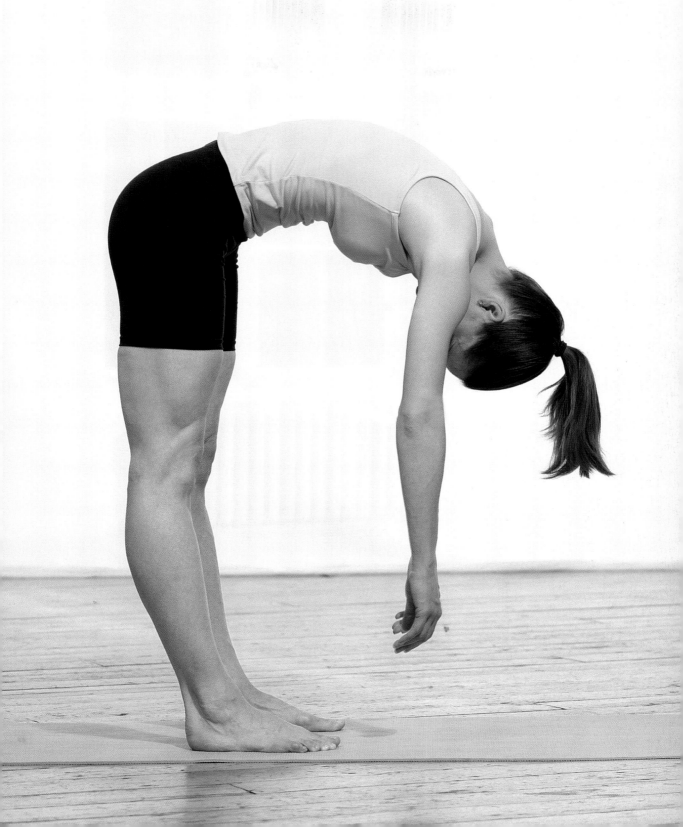

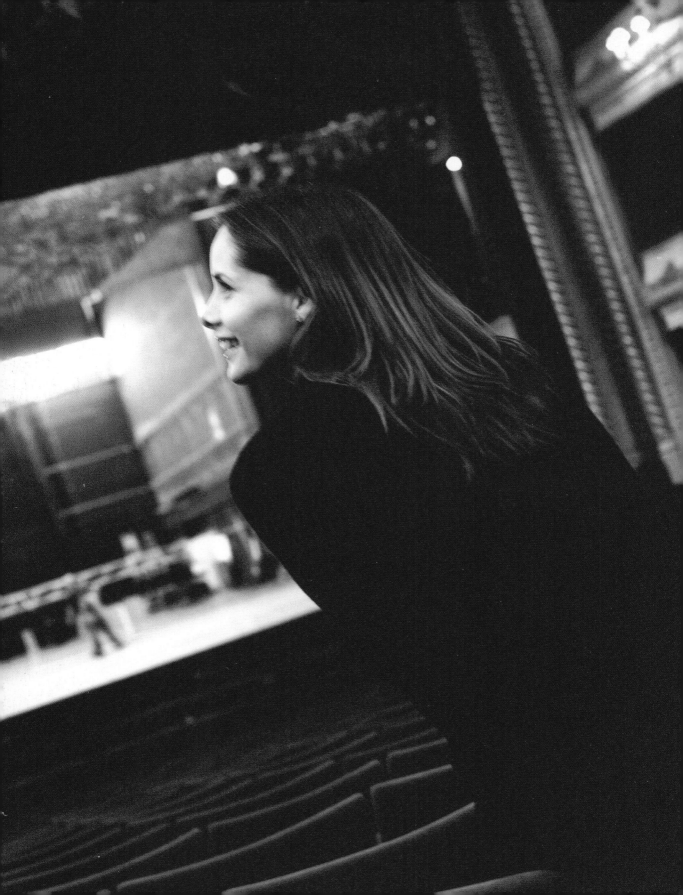

WARM UP / FLEXIBILITY

Don't be tempted to skip this section. It's very important always to warm your body up before doing the exercise programme. You can injure yourself and are more likely to carry out the exercises incorrectly if your muscles aren't stretched and warm before you begin.

Ideally, even when you're not doing the Pilates core programme, you should do some gentle stretching every day. This will help improve your flexibility, which in turn means your joints and muscles will be more mobile when you exercise. As you get older, your muscles lose their elasticity and you become less supple, so the importance and benefit of doing regular and frequent stretches increases, otherwise your muscles could become tighter and tighter.

Be careful though not to warm up either half-heartedly or for too long – ten minutes is enough. Warm ups are all about gently moving your body and doing circles of your joints to prepare for the real exercise, so jogging on the spot is excellent for example, as are the exercises in this section. Obviously don't just get out of bed and jump around madly the first time you try this. The key is to be gentle and do natural stretches that suit your body – so don't move beyond your range or force yourself into positions that feel painful or too uncomfortable. Also remember to breathe into the stretches as this helps you to hold the position and lengthen into them.

seated roll down

1 Sit upright on a chair or on your bed with your feet firmly on the floor, parallel and hip-width apart. Gently draw your belly button towards your spine – this activates your stomach muscles and helps you sit up straight.

2 Inhale, and on the exhale drop your chin to your chest and roll your body down, imagining each individual vertebra moving as you go (you may not be able to roll down that far to start with).

3 When you can go no further, inhale; then uncurl slowly and return to the starting position.

Repeat ten times.

The focus with this exercise is on waking up the spine and moving it vertebra by vertebra to open out and stretch the back.

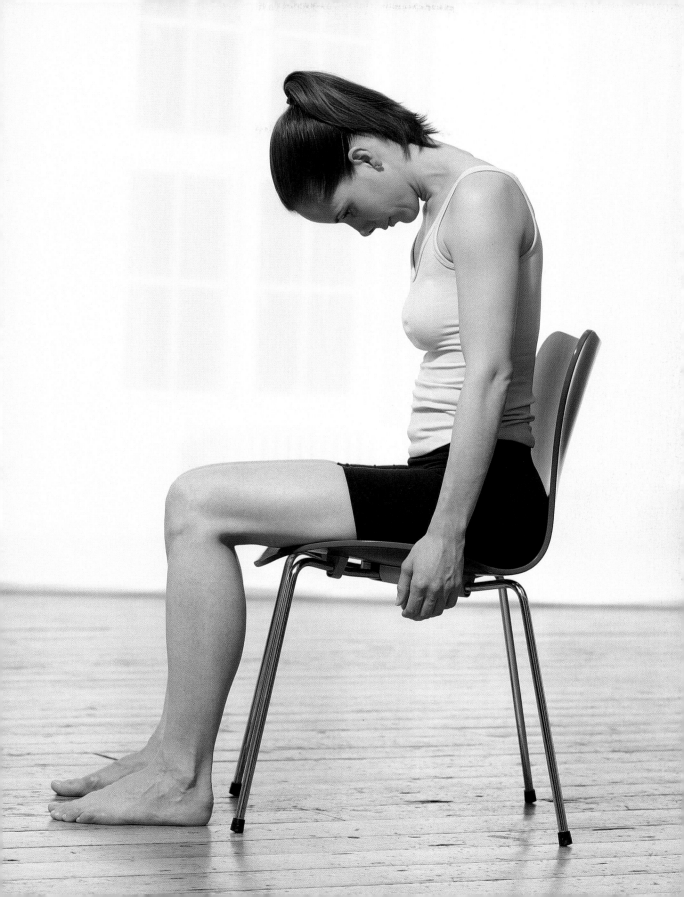

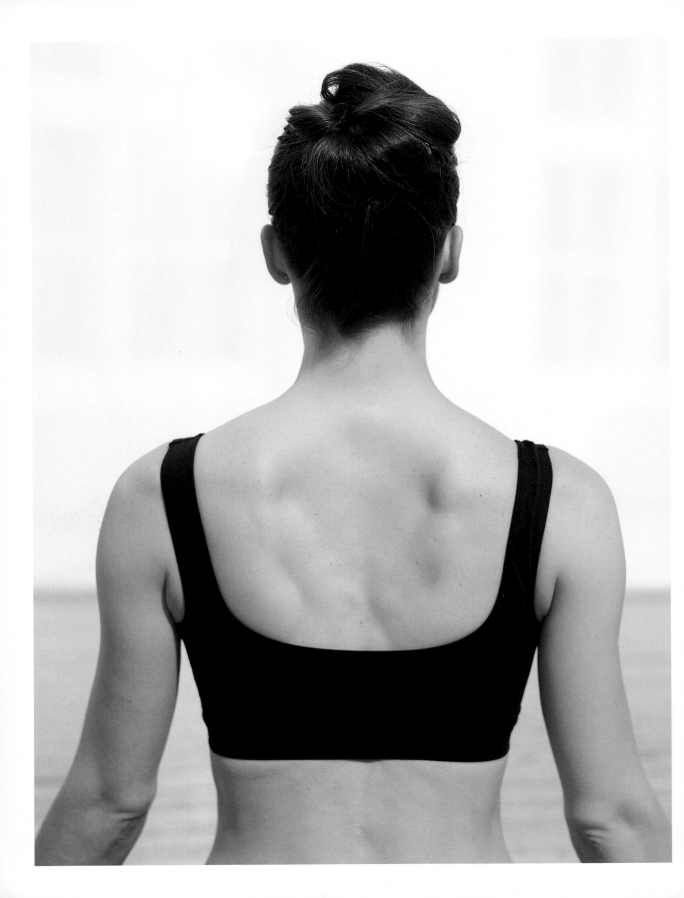

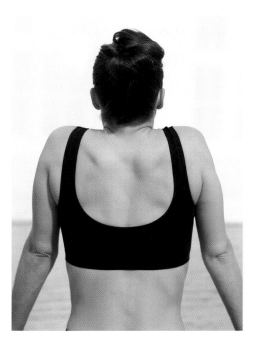 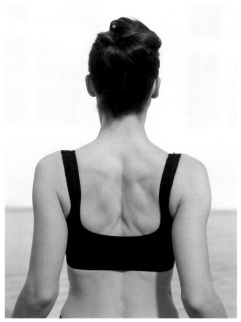

shoulder rolls

1   Standing tall, have your arms resting gently at your sides.

2   Lift both your shoulders to your ears and roll them backwards, completing a full rotation until they are back at the starting position. Breathe normally as you do this and be sure to drop your shoulder blades as you move. Repeat the action, but this time move your shoulders forwards.

Do ten rolls in one direction and then ten in the other.

Most of us walk round with our shoulders hunched up. This exercise helps to mobilize the shoulders and loosen the upper back.

neck stretches (I)

1 Sit upright on the floor with your stomach pulled in, and tuck your chin into your neck (so you have a double chin).

2 Inhale and drop your chin to your chest. Exhale and hold for ten seconds. You should feel the stretch down the back of your neck and spine.

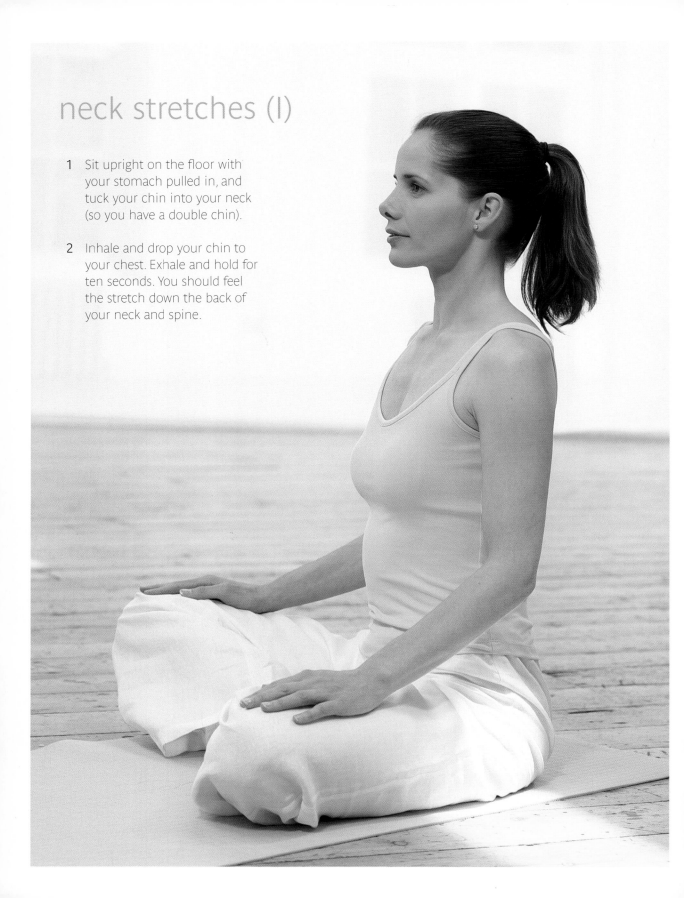

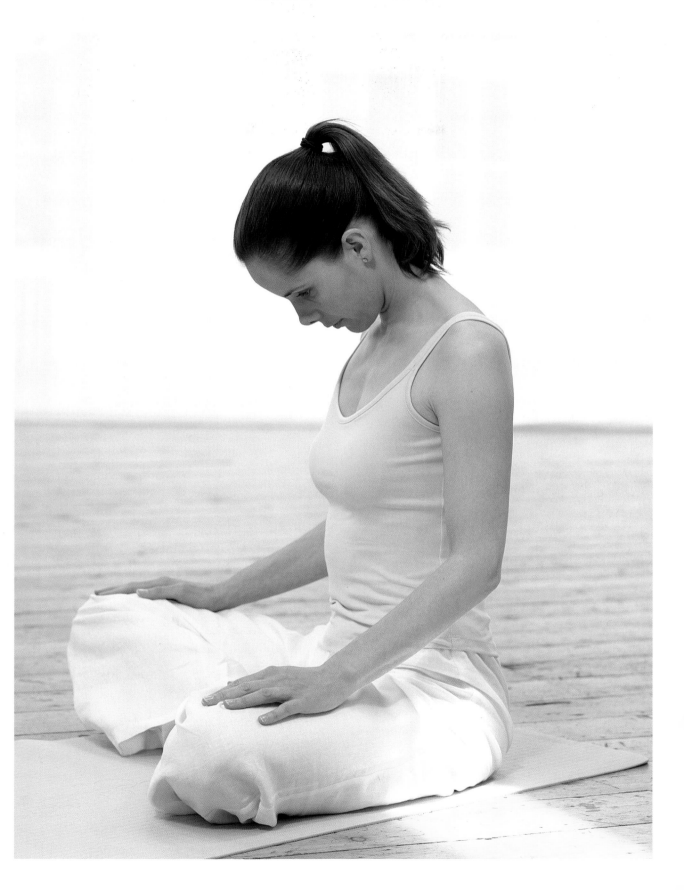

neck stretches (II)

1   Sitting upright on the floor
with your stomach pulled in,
inhale and drop your head over
to the left, exhale and hold for
ten seconds (you should feel
the stretch down the right side
of your neck and spine).

2   Return to the starting position
and repeat on the other side.

Repeat three times on each
side, alternating between them.

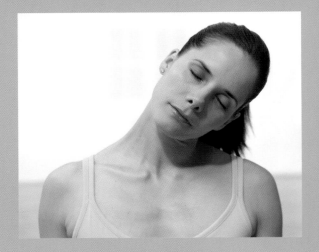

TIP

AS A PROGRESSION,
WHEN YOU DROP
YOUR HEAD OVER TO
THE LEFT, PLACE YOUR
LEFT HAND OVER
YOUR RIGHT EAR AND
LET THE WEIGHT
OF YOUR HAND PULL
YOUR HEAD TOWARDS
YOUR SHOULDER.
REPEAT ON THE
OTHER SIDE.

A great stretch for anyone who
has to sit at a desk all day or
who has a stiff neck and
shoulders.

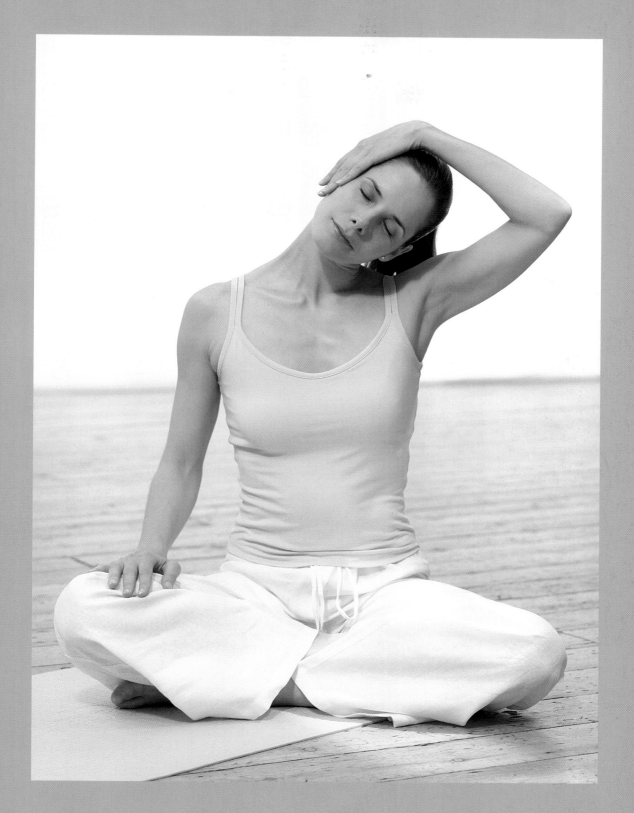

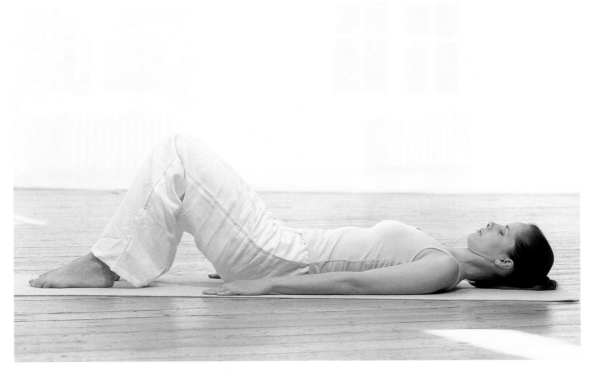

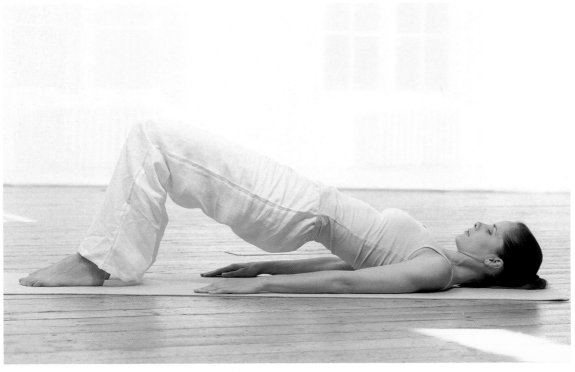

bridging

1 Lie on your back with your knees bent at a ninety-degree angle, feet in parallel and hip-width apart, and your arms by your sides.

2 Exhale and engage your pelvic floor, stomach and bottom muscles, slowly peeling your spine off the mat, one vertebra at a time, until your hips are in line with your knees.

3 Inhale and hold your body perfectly still.

4 Exhale and, using your stomach muscles, slowly roll down through your spine, lowering one vertebra at a time. Keep your bottom up until the last minute and then let it sink into the floor.

Repeat ten times.

A basic lower-back warm-up exercise that will awaken your spine.

pelvic clock

1 This is an exercise where you don't physically move, but where you need to imagine the movement. Start by lying on the floor on your back with your knees bent at a ninety-degree angle, feet in parallel and hip-width apart, and arms by your sides.

2 Inhale and visualize one of your hips moving up towards the belly button, around to the other side and down to the pubic bone. Once you get the sensation, speed it up for ten repetitions.

3 Eventually, after doing this exercise a number of times, you will feel movement in these muscles without actually moving your body.

Repeat on the other side for ten repetitions.

You may not feel it does anything, but this is a very strong exercise for your stomach muscles.

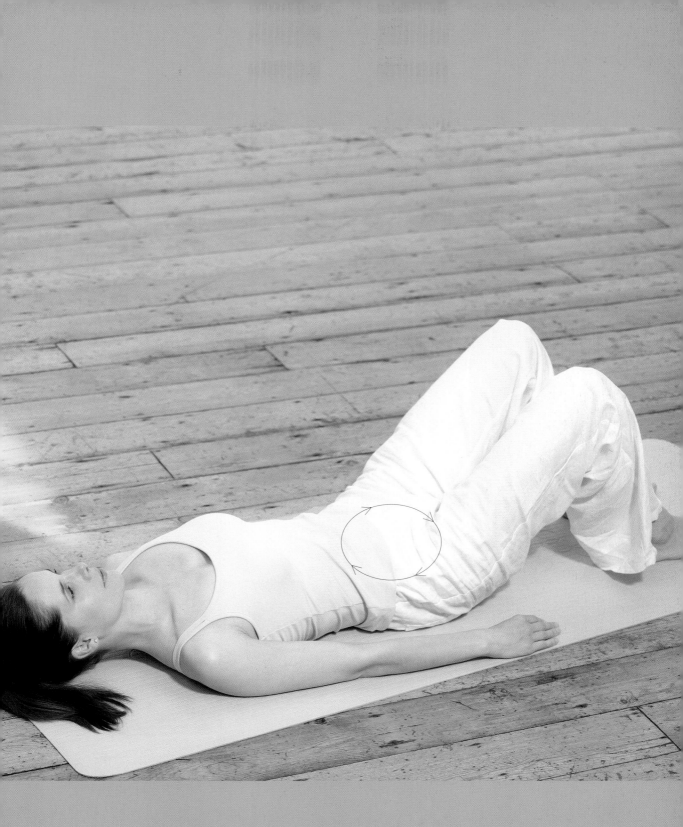

knees to chest stretch

1 Lie on your back with your knees together and bent at a ninety-degree angle. Place a cushion under your bottom and lift your knees to your chest holding them in place with your hands. Your bottom should be just resting on the cushion.

2 Inhale and slowly draw your knees to your chest, pulling your stomach in at the same time.

3 To help stretch your spine more, exhale and imagine your tailbone lengthening away from your head.

4 Inhale and relax your spine, letting your tailbone drop back on to the cushion.

Repeat five times.

A lovely lower-back stretch.

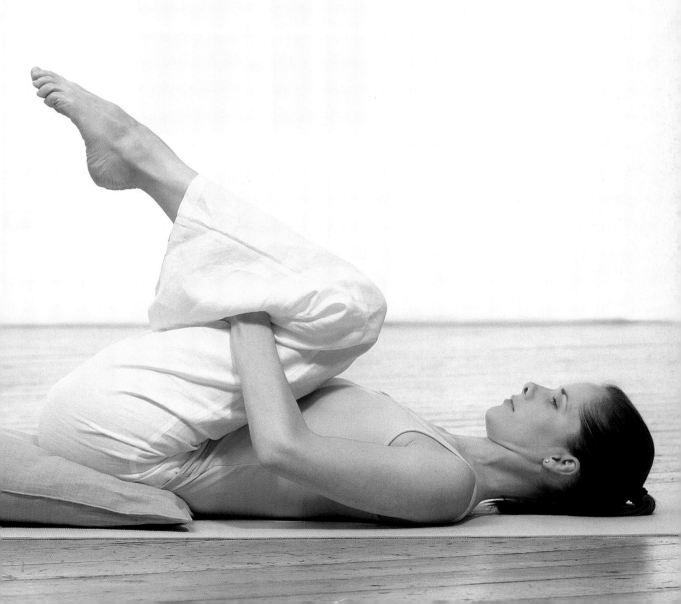

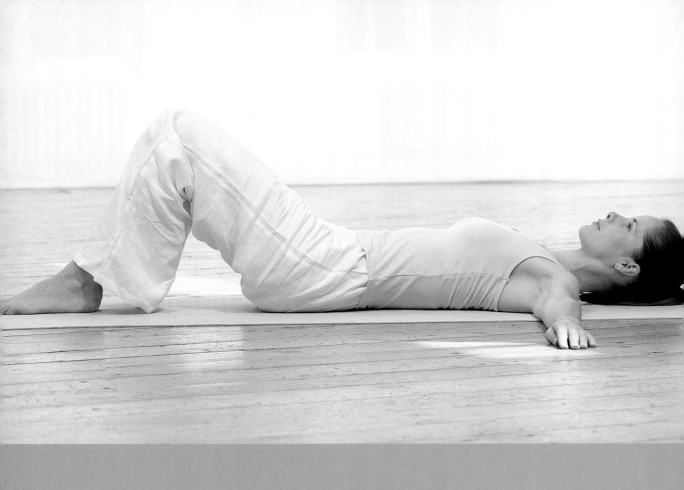

Your obliques – the side stomach muscles – are often underworked so this exercise is perfect if you want a toned waist.

knee rolling (I)

1 Lie on your back with your knees together and bent at a ninety-degree angle.

2 Stretch your arms out to the sides at shoulder height (don't let your shoulders rise to your ears).

3 As you inhale pull your stomach in, and, using your stomach muscles, roll your knees to one side, ensuring you keep your opposing hip fixed to the floor. Don't try to force your legs all the way down to the floor.

4 As you exhale, use your stomach muscles to move your legs back to the starting position and repeat on the other side.

Repeat five times on each side, alternating between them.

knee rolling (II)

An excellent progression
from the first knee-rolling
exercise that brings in
inner-thigh work.

1 Lie on your back with your
knees bent and place a cushion
between them. Hold it there as
you lift your legs off the floor
to a ninety-degree angle so
your knees end up over your
hips. Use your inner thighs to
hold the cushion in place.

2 Stretch your arms out to the
sides at shoulder height. As you
inhale, pull your stomach in,
and use your stomach muscles
to roll your knees to one side
(you may not get very far),
keeping your opposing hip
fixed to the floor.

3 As you exhale, use your
stomach muscles to return to
the starting position. Repeat on
the other side, being sure to
control the movement and
keeping your spine fixed.

Repeat five times on each side,
alternating between them.

TIP

BE CAREFUL TO AVOID
A BUNCHED STOMACH.

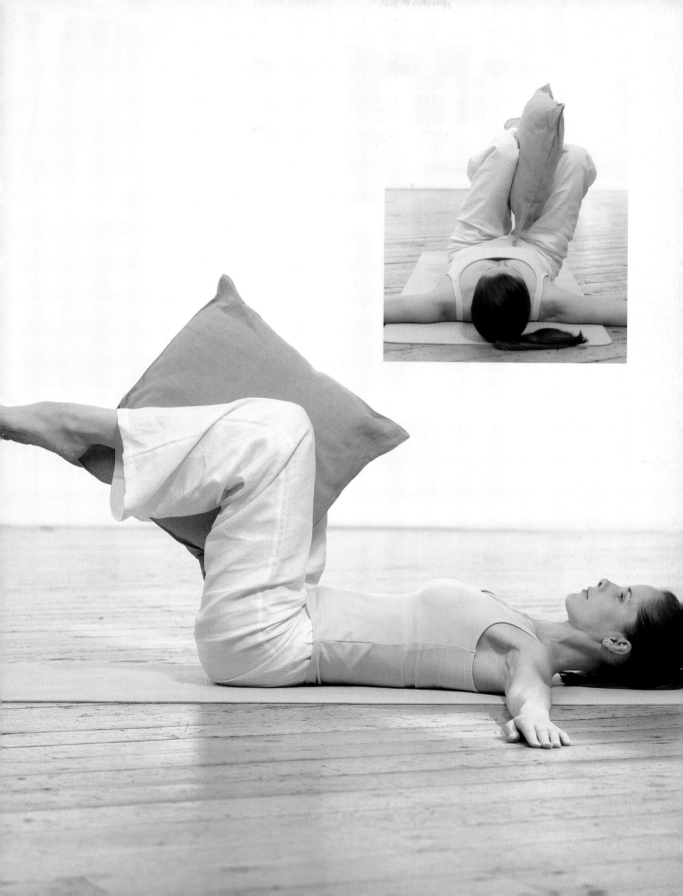

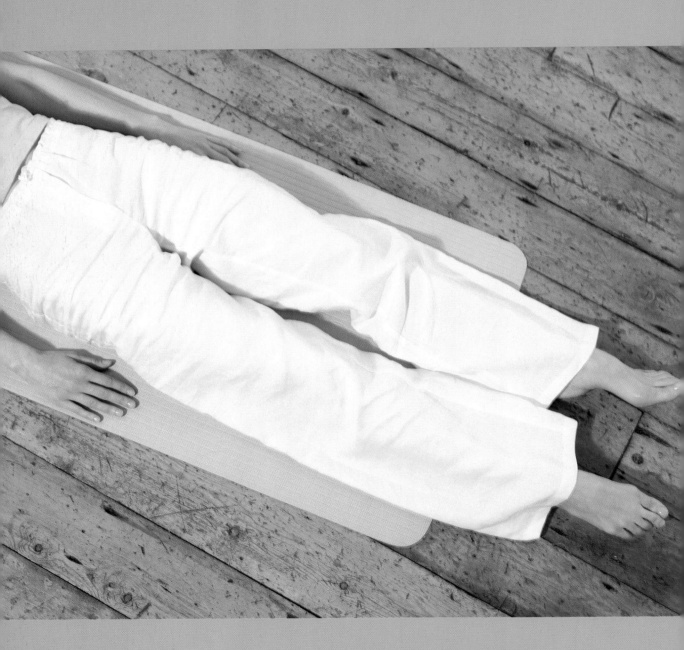

hip hitching

1 Lie on the floor on your back. Your legs should be straight and hip-width apart. Have your arms by your sides and your stomach pulled in.

2 Keeping your legs on the floor, hitch up one hip and at the same time stretch out your other leg (imagine your leg pulling away from your hip joint) and extend your foot towards the wall in front of you. The legs work in opposition here. As one leg hitches up, the opposing leg lengthens down.

3 Exhale and return to the starting position. Repeat on the other side.

Repeat five times on each leg, alternating between them.

This exercise lengthens your hips and gives a good pull on your spine.

> **TIP**
>
> BE SURE TO KEEP YOUR RIBS DROPPED AND YOUR UPPER BODY RELAXED.

spine stretch

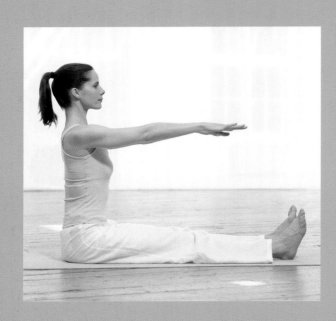

1   Sit up straight with your legs extended in front of you, your feet slightly wider than hip-width apart and flexed.

2   Lift your arms straight out in front of you at shoulder height. Inhale and drop your chin to your chest, rounding your back and pulling your belly button towards your spine. Imagine you are in a giant C-shape.

3   Exhale and stretch your arms forwards towards your feet (keep your hips stable). You may not be able to go that far to begin with but you will progress.

4   Inhale and reverse the motion, rolling back up from a C-shape to your original position.

Repeat five times.

> **TIP**
>
> IMAGINE YOU'RE CURVING YOUR UPPER BODY OVER A LARGE BEACH BALL THAT'S RESTING ON YOUR THIGHS, AND THEN ROLLING BACK UP AGAINST A WALL.

This is a wonderful hamstring stretch and a good progression exercise because eventually your hands will go past your toes.

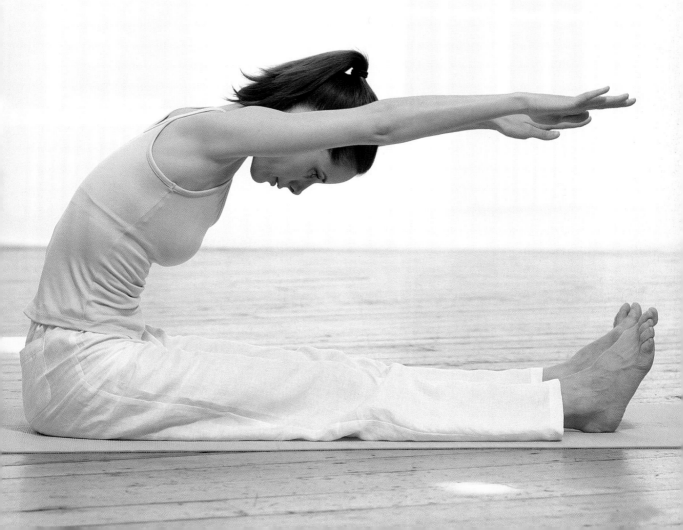

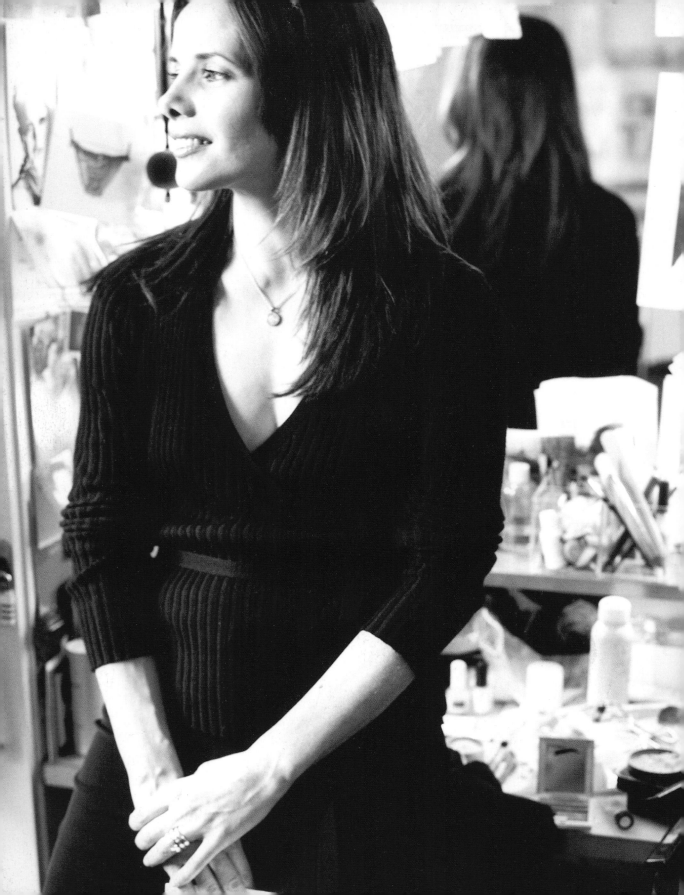

MAIN PROGRAMME

Anyone who does Pilates wants to get a flat stomach and this is one of the great benefits of this technique. All the exercises in this section will help you achieve this goal. Go to any gym and you'll see lots of people doing sit-ups because they think this is the right way to get a flat stomach, but they're wrong. With sit-ups all you're doing is building a bulk of bunched-up muscle in your abdomen which makes your stomach stick out more – this is why sit-ups don't work.

In Pilates you do the opposite. The exercises work your deep postural muscles known as transversus abdominis. These run around the body like a corset and research shows that building these muscles creates what's known as core stability, which helps you look taller, flatter and straighter.

To engage the abdominal muscles don't imagine bunching them up tightly, instead, pull your belly button to your spine and then 'scoop' your abdominals upwards to make your stomach look really flat and lengthened. If there's any kind of bulge or you're getting any kind of pain in your back or your stomach you're not doing it right; focus on keeping your stomach muscles pulled in and up.

The good thing is that once you know how to engage your abdominals you can work them anywhere – while waiting for a bus or queuing at the bank. Just pull your belly button towards your spine, drop your ribs and shoulders and breathe with them held in. No one will notice, so you can do as many repetitions as you like and hold it for as long as you like.

abdominals

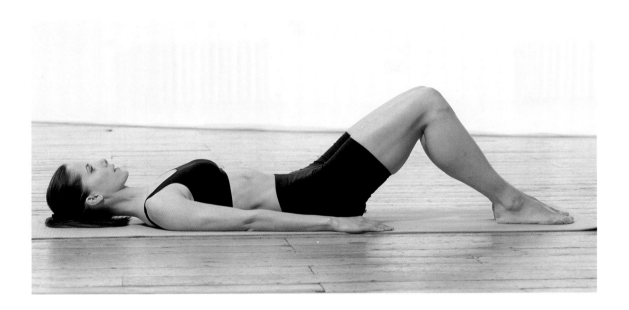

bent-knee fall-outs

These are my favourites as they are easy to do, but incredibly effective as a lower abdominal workout.

1. Lie on the floor with your knees bent at a ninety-degree angle, feet parallel and hip-width apart, your belly button pulled towards your spine and your arms by your sides.

2. Inhale, and as you exhale let one of your knees fall outwards in a controlled movement towards the floor, making sure your other leg doesn't fall in and your hips and pelvis don't move or waver. You should feel a stretch in your lower abdominals on the opposing side as the knee falls out.

3. Inhale and at the same time use your stomach muscles to return to the starting position. Repeat on the other side.

Repeat five times on each leg, alternating between them.

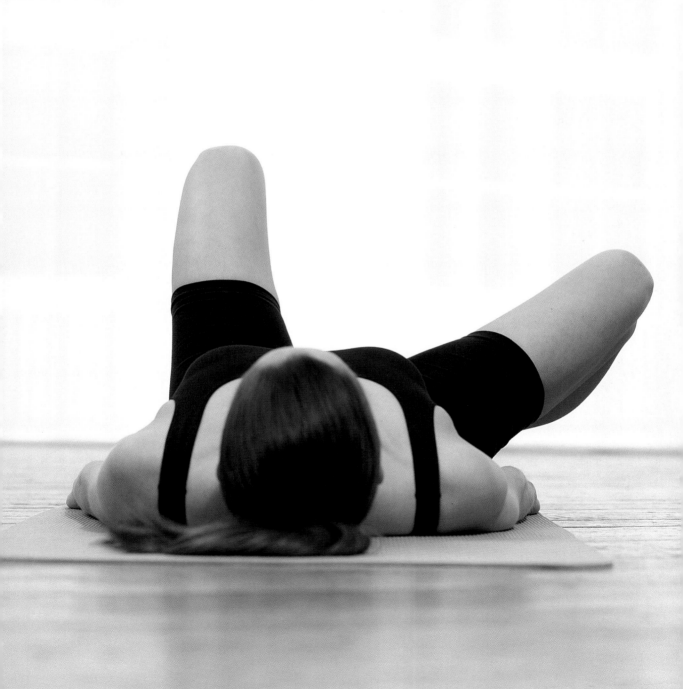

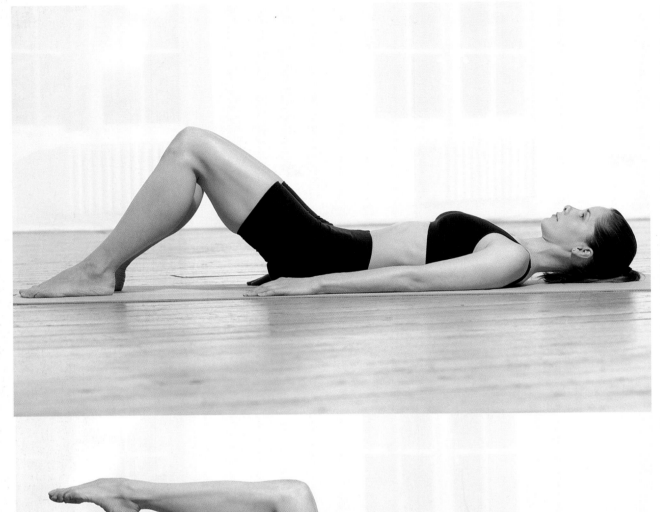

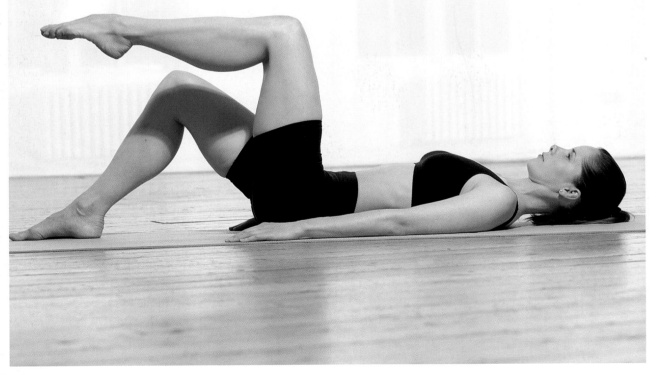

single leg raise

1   Lie on the floor with your knees bent at a ninety-degree angle, feet parallel and hip-width apart, your belly button pulled towards your spine and your arms by your sides.

2   Slowly inhale and at the same time pull your stomach muscles in and let one leg float up off the floor bringing the knee over the hip, keeping your leg at a ninety-degree angle. Hold for two counts, and on the exhale return your leg to the floor in two counts.

Repeat ten times on each leg, alternating between them.

I call this a cleaning-your-teeth exercise because it can be done every day and it's one of the best stomach-awakening exercises.

double leg raise

1   Lie on the floor with your
knees bent at a ninety-degree
angle, feet parallel and hip-
width apart, your belly button
pulled towards your spine and
your arms by your sides.

2   Slowly pull your stomach
muscles in, breathing normally,
then let one leg float up until
the knee is over the hip,
keeping your leg at a ninety-
degree angle. Then bring your
other leg up to the same
position and hold for two
counts. Allow the first leg to go
back down in two counts and
then the other. Control both
your legs on the way down to
the floor with your stomach
muscles; don't push down
with your hands.

Repeat ten times.

The crucial point to
remember here is that when
you bring your legs up, your
spine should be in neutral so
that your core muscles are
doing all the hard work.

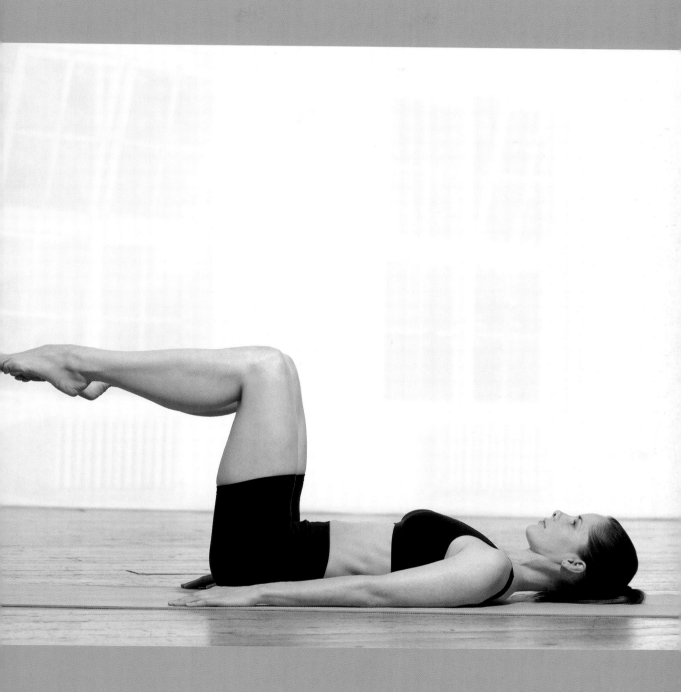

bugs (I)

1 Lie on the floor with your knees bent at a ninety-degree angle, feet parallel and hip-width apart, your belly button pulled towards your spine and your arms by your sides.

2 Inhale and slide one leg along the floor as your opposing arm rises and extends behind your head. Make sure your shoulders don't rise when you do this.

3 Hold for two counts, exhale, and return to the starting position. Repeat on the other side.

Repeat five times on each side, alternating between them.

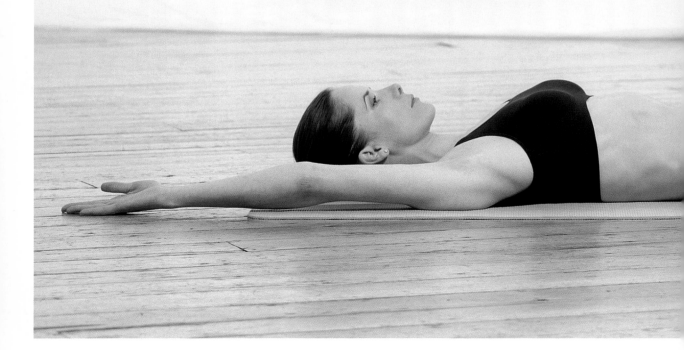

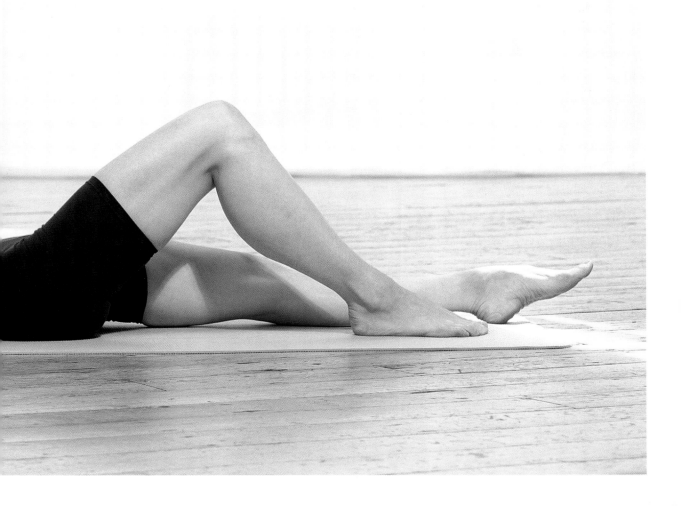

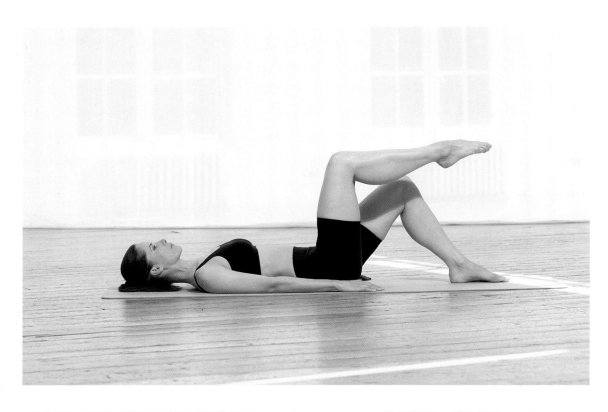

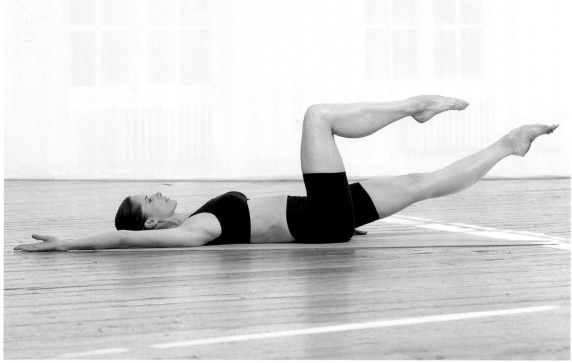

bugs (II)

1   Lie on the floor with one knee bent and the other lifted off the floor so your knee is over the hip and at a ninety-degree angle. Keep your arms by your sides.

2   Inhale and slide the foot on the floor forwards so the leg extends fully, then lift it off the floor slightly. At the same time extend your opposing arm by lifting it above and behind your head. Make sure your shoulders don't rise when you do this.

3   Hold for two counts, exhale, and come back to the starting position. Repeat on the other side.

Repeat five times on each side, alternating between them.

These two exercises are the perfect way to lengthen and stretch the body.

Having strong upper-
stomach muscles is very
important because it
helps you maintain
posture and alignment
at all times.

curl ups (modified)

1　Lie on the floor with your knees
bent at a ninety-degree angle,
feet parallel and hip-width
apart. Place your hands behind
your head.

2　Inhale and at the same time
pull in your abdominals and
curl your head and chest off the
floor. Keeping your elbows wide,
aim your gaze at your knees to
align your head and engage
your core. Make sure you don't
pull your head forwards with
your hands or initiate the
movement with your hip
flexors.

3　Exhale and slowly curl back
down to the floor.

Repeat five times.

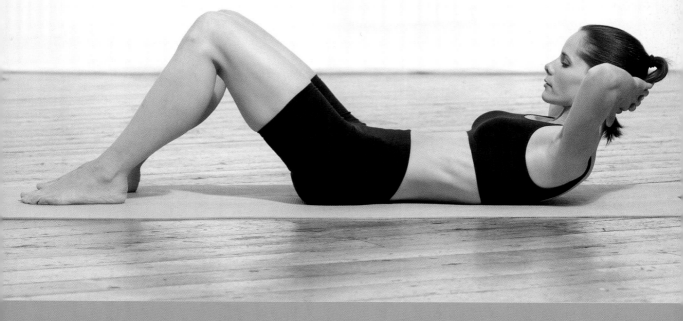

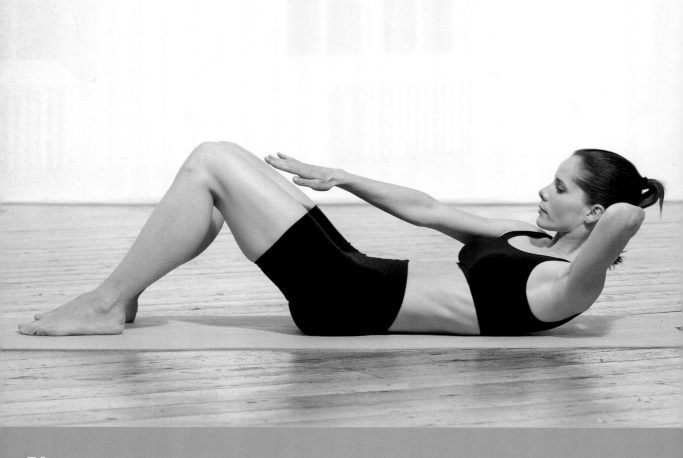

obliques (modified)

1 Lie on the floor with your knees bent at a ninety-degree angle, feet parallel and hip-width apart. Place one hand behind your head and the other by your side. Inhale.

2 As you exhale, scoop in your abdominals and curl your head and chest off the floor (fix your gaze on your knees), and twist as you move your free arm towards your opposing knee.

3 Exhale and slowly curl back down to the floor and repeat with your other arm.

Repeat five times on each side, alternating between them.

Obliques are your side abdominal muscles, which lie around your waist. This exercise will work your waist and your stomach at the same time.

hundreds

This is a staple of any Pilates programme. It's a very good exercise because as you advance you'll quickly see the improvement.

1 Lie on the floor with your legs together and lifted, so your knees are above your hips and at a ninety-degree angle. Keep your arms by your sides.

2 Lift your head and upper body and aim your gaze towards your belly button to engage your stomach muscles.

3 Stretch your arms forwards and lift them slightly off the floor (imagine your fingers stretching away from you). Keeping your arms straight, start pumping them up and down in a steady rhythm, breathing normally as you do this.

4 Continue for a minimum of ten counts, but aim for a hundred if you can.

TIP

MAKE SURE YOUR SHOULDERS ARE STABILIZED AND PART OF YOUR BLADES ARE PRESSED TO THE GROUND.

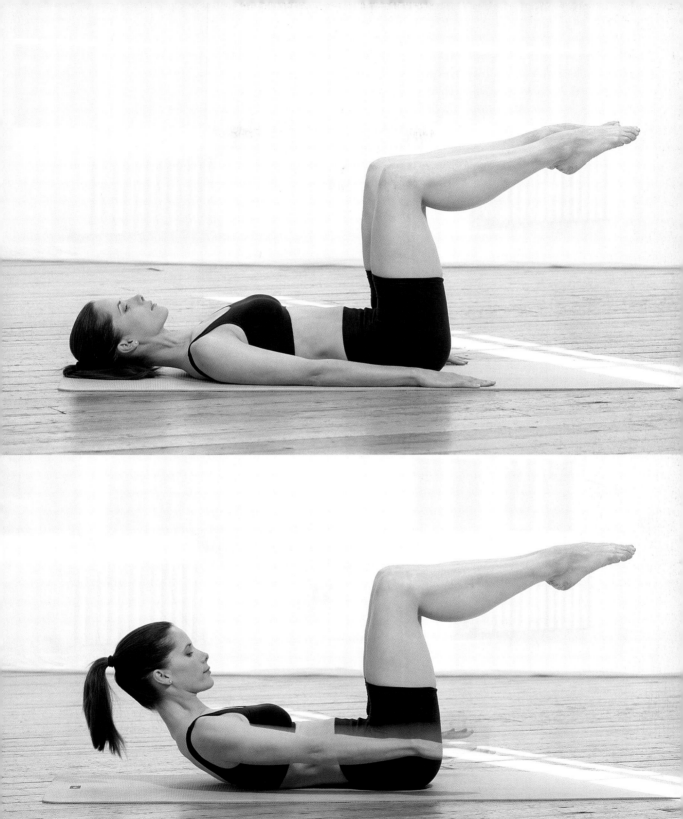

criss cross

1 Lie on the floor with your knees bent and together above your hips at a ninety-degree angle. Place your hands behind your head.

2 Inhale and, pulling your abdominals in, curl your head and chest off the floor, being sure that you don't pull your head forwards with your hands. Aim your right elbow at your left knee, at the same time extending the right leg, pushing through the toe. Keep your left leg bent.

3 Exhale and come back to centre, keeping your head lifted. Repeat on the opposite side.

Repeat five times on each side, alternating between them.

TIP

MOST PEOPLE FIND THIS EXERCISE DIFFICULT TO BEGIN WITH, BUT IT PAYS TO PERSEVERE.

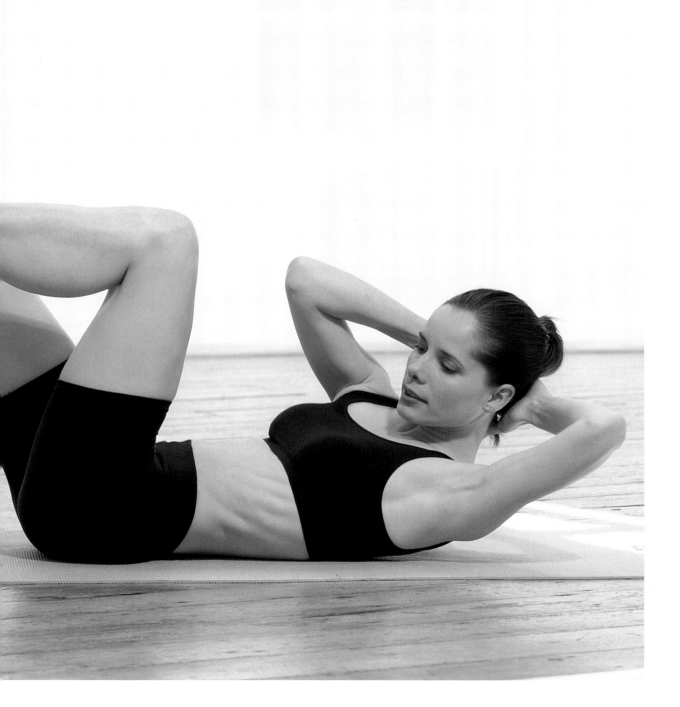

The aim of stretching is to increase your flexibility, but it is also very important because it helps prevent injury and reduces post-exercise stiffness. During any type of exercise muscles shorten and become tight and hard. When you stretch you are trying to increase the range of muscle movement around a joint or joints that may feel stiff.

To stretch effectively, make sure you move slowly into the position and then hold for thirty seconds. Always breathe slowly and deeply when holding the stretch and, for maximum effect, focus on the muscle, imagining it lengthening. Never bounce when stretching as this can lead to injury. Finally, always move slowly out of a stretch and relax for a few minutes before continuing your exercise programme.

When you stretch, there may be a small amount of pain. The pain however should be a dull one that lessens as you breathe through it. If you ever feel a sharp pain when stretching, stop immediately.

stretching

glute stretch

1   Lie on your back with your knees bent and place your right ankle across the left knee.

2   Lifting your head up clasp your hands around your left thigh. Inhale and pull your knee towards you (at the same time return your head to the floor).

3   Exhale and slowly pull your knee towards your chest. You should feel a stretch across your glutes (bottom). Hold for thirty seconds and release.

Repeat four times on one leg and then four times on the other.

Don't be alarmed if one side is tighter than the other. This is completely normal.

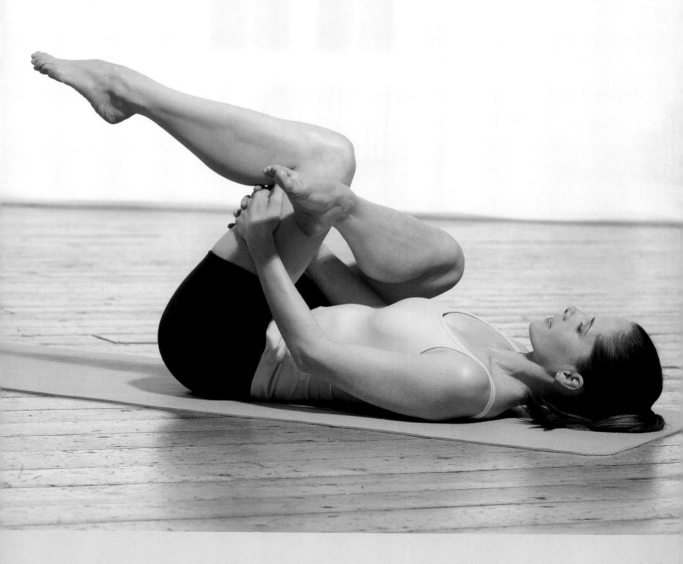

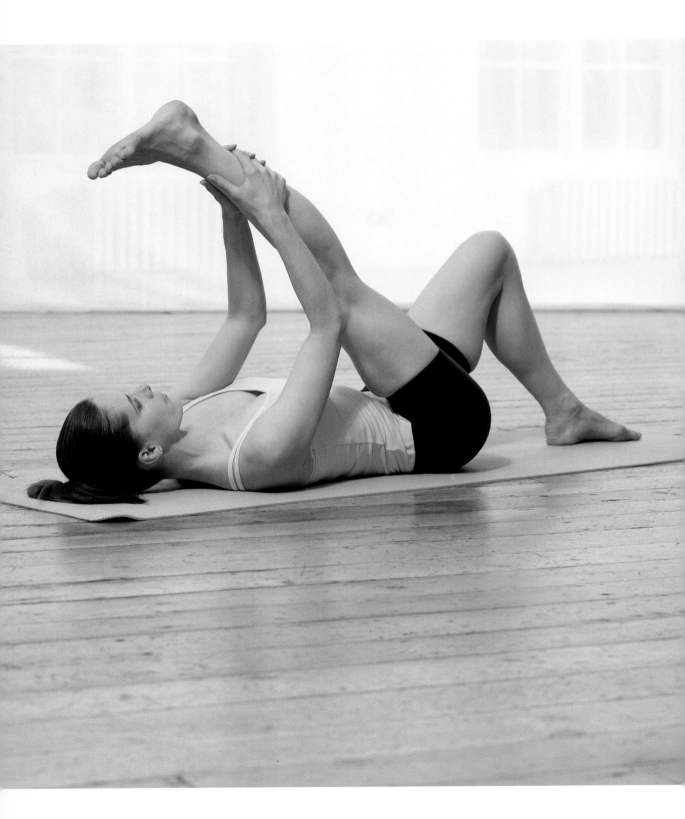

hamstrings

1 Lie down on the floor with your knees bent at a ninety-degree angle. Lift one leg into the air so it's straight, then clasp your hands around the back of your knee.

2 Inhaling, gently pull your leg towards you, making sure it stays straight and your bottom and hips remain on the ground. You should feel the stretch from your bottom towards your knee. Hold for thirty seconds.

3 Exhale and return your leg to the starting position. Repeat on the other leg.

Repeat five times on one leg and then five times on the other.

This is one to do every day because if your hamstrings are unduly tight you may suffer from back problems. Don't worry if to begin with you can't pull your leg close to your body. Over time your hamstring muscles will become more supple and you'll have greater flexibility.

TIP

FOR A FULL RANGE OF MOVEMENT, IMAGINE YOUR LEG SINKING DOWN INTO YOUR HIP JOINT AS YOU PULL IT TOWARDS YOU.

frogs

1 Sit upright on the floor and place the soles of your feet together.

2 Holding your ankles, slide the heels of your feet towards your bottom, so that your knees are bent outwards in a frog-like position.

3 Breathing normally, hold for thirty seconds.

4 To increase the stretch bring the feet closer to your body.

Works the inner thighs to help tone them up.

TIP

DON'T TRY TO GET YOUR KNEES ONTO THE GROUND THE FIRST TIME. EVENTUALLY YOU'LL BECOME MORE FLEXIBLE AND YOUR KNEES WILL DROP.

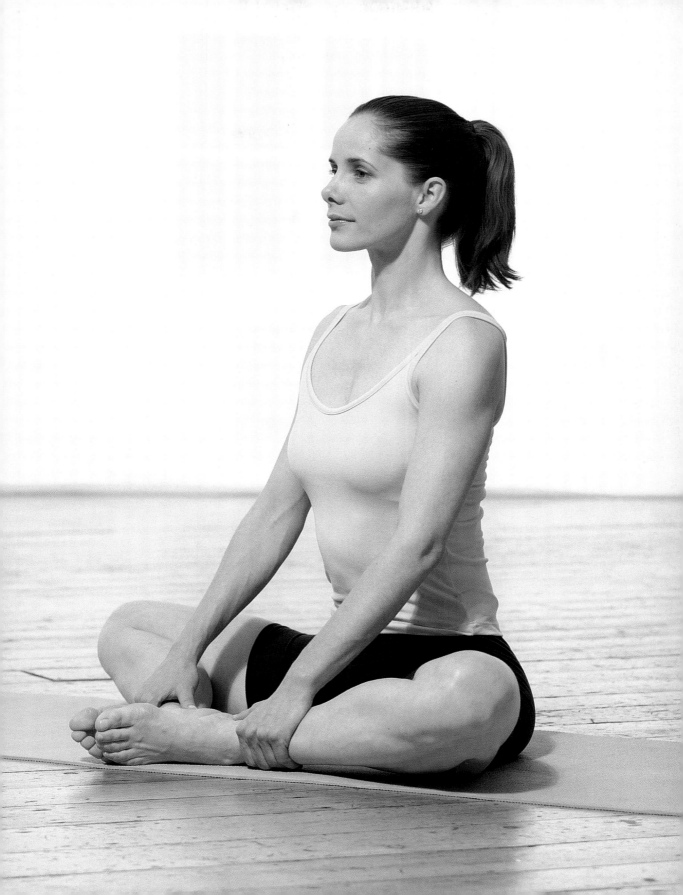

These seated exercises are good for people who have to sit at a desk all day, because they ensure you stay strong and mobile and help you achieve a better posture. Sedentary jobs and lifestyles mean your back and stomach muscles become severely underused, and in many cases the stomach muscles cannot then support the abdomen, so the spine takes over and takes all the strain. If you spend a large part of your day sitting, these exercises are invaluable for preventing back pain as you get older.

A classic bad standing or sitting stance is to suck your stomach in, pull yourself straight, puff out your chest and let your chin poke out. If this sounds familiar, it's worth noting that the spine is not naturally straight and the best way to sit is with a gentle natural curve in the small of your back. Think tall, keep feet hip-width apart and imagine there is a string pulling you up from the centre of your head. At the same time, make sure your head is aligned with your spine and tuck your chin in (as if you were going for a double chin).

Perfect these seated exercises and they will help you think about how you do everyday things such as sitting, standing and bending; you will learn not to throw yourself into a chair when you sit down, or brace yourself when you get up. Other tips include pulling down the muscles under your shoulders to let your shoulders roll back, and, when you're sitting, to ensure your legs aren't crossed and you're supporting yourself from your stomach, not sinking into your waist.

sitting

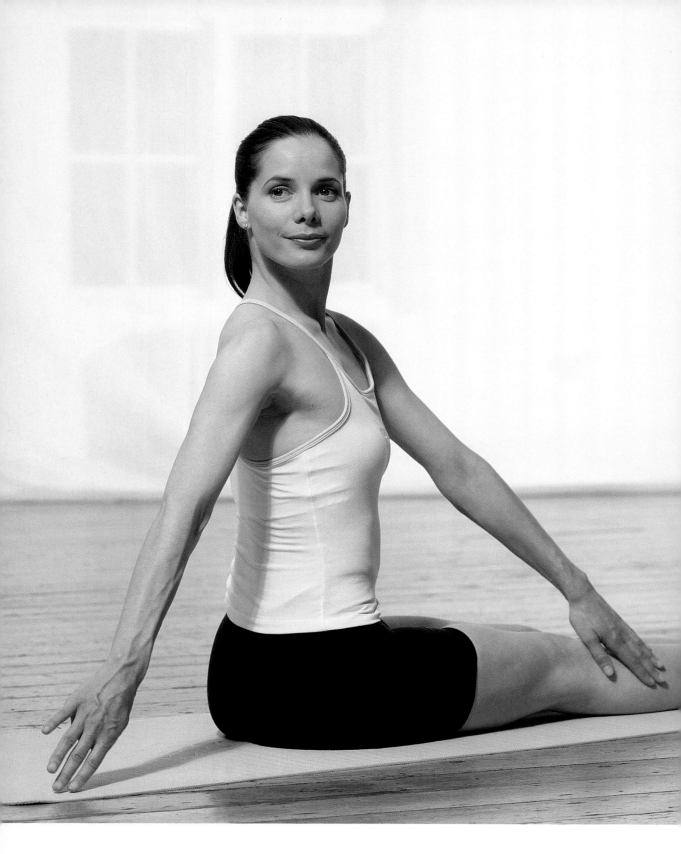

spine twist

1 Sit upright on the floor, lifting up from your abdominals (imagine you are sitting straight against a wall). Keep your legs straight in front of you and hip-width apart with your feet flexed.

2 With your arms stretched out in front of you, keeping your hips stationary, inhale and twist from the waist to the right, letting your arms swing down to your sides. Hold for one count.

3 Exhale and come back to the starting position, then twist in the opposite direction.

Repeat five times on each side, alternating between them.

Works your obliques and wittles down your waist.

TIP

DO NOT FORCE THIS MOVEMENT; JUST TURN AS FAR AS YOU CAN TO FEEL A COMPLETE STRETCH WHILE BEING CAREFUL NOT TO LEAN BACK.

the saw

1 Sit upright on the floor, lifting up from your abdominals (imagine you are sitting straight against a wall). Position your legs straight in front of you in a wide V-shape and keep your feet flexed.

2 Keeping your arms parallel to the floor, extend them out to the side. Inhale and twist your upper body to the left, then slowly dive forwards, aiming your right arm towards your left foot.

3 Exhale, then inhale and draw your stomach in, returning to the upright position. Repeat on the other side.

Repeat three times on each side, alternating between them.

A good exercise as it incorporates an abdominal twist with a hamstring stretch.

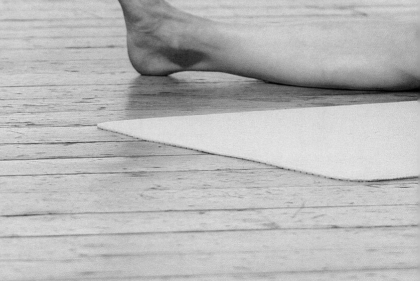

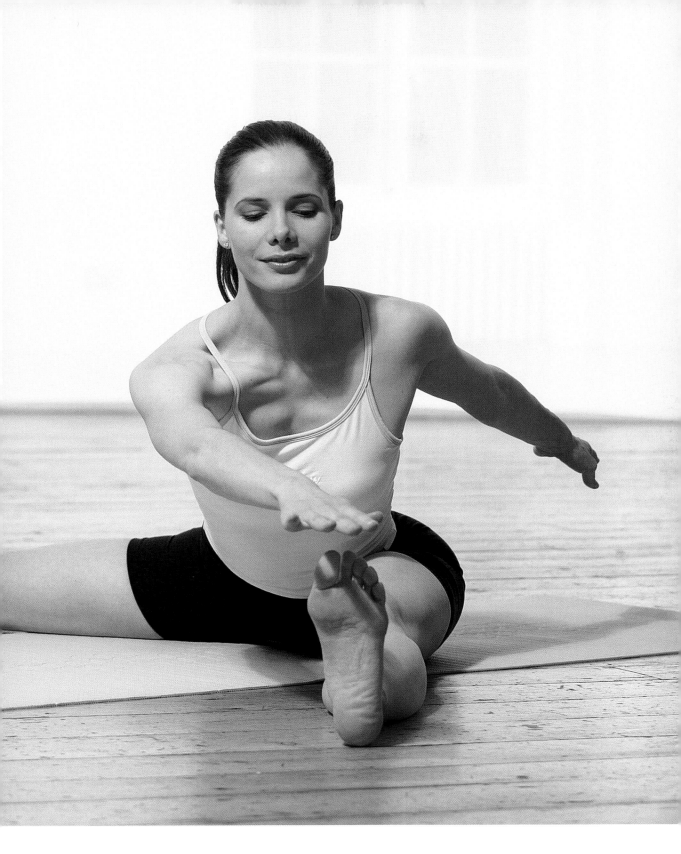

The kneeling Pilates positions are all about stability and strengthening your back, which again means focusing on your core muscles. In theory, we should use our stomach muscles for everything; if we did, there would be far less back pain or hamstring problems. That's why the core is so important.

The aim of the four-point kneeling exercises is to isolate certain muscles. It is important you always work both sides of your body to even yourself out; we all have one side that's definitely weaker than the other. (You will usually be stronger on the right if you are right-handed and vice versa; if this is marked, do two repetitions on one side and one on the other.)

Whatever you do, don't push yourself too far — if you're sweating and killing yourself you're putting too much effort into it. Pilates is a gentle form of exercise: you don't push into the movements or force anything. You certainly shouldn't experience any sharp pains when you do them. Always begin moderately and recognize your limitations; you will then experience a great sense of satisfaction as your body tones, tightens and strengthens.

four-point kneeling

dog

1. Get onto all fours on the floor. Knees should be under hips, arms under shoulders and head aligned with your back in a straight line, with your stomach pulled in and shoulders pulled down.

2. Breathing normally, lift one leg off the floor and, keeping it bent at ninety degrees, extend your foot to the ceiling, bringing your knee in line with your hip. Then return it to the starting position.

   Repeat five times on each leg, alternating between them.

TIP

MAKE SURE YOU KEEP YOUR BACK STRAIGHT AND DON'T LET YOUR SHOULDER BLADES SINK IN.

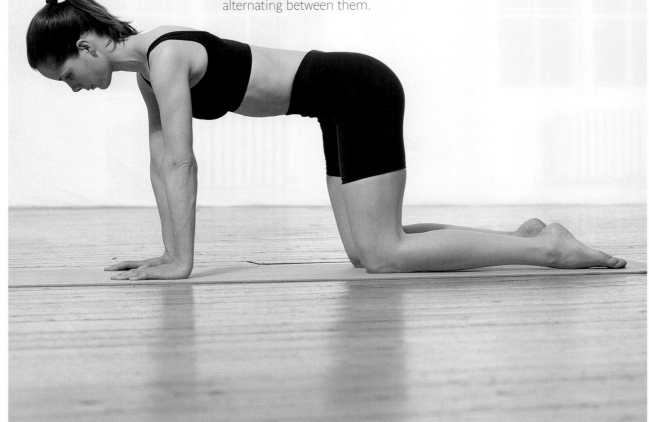

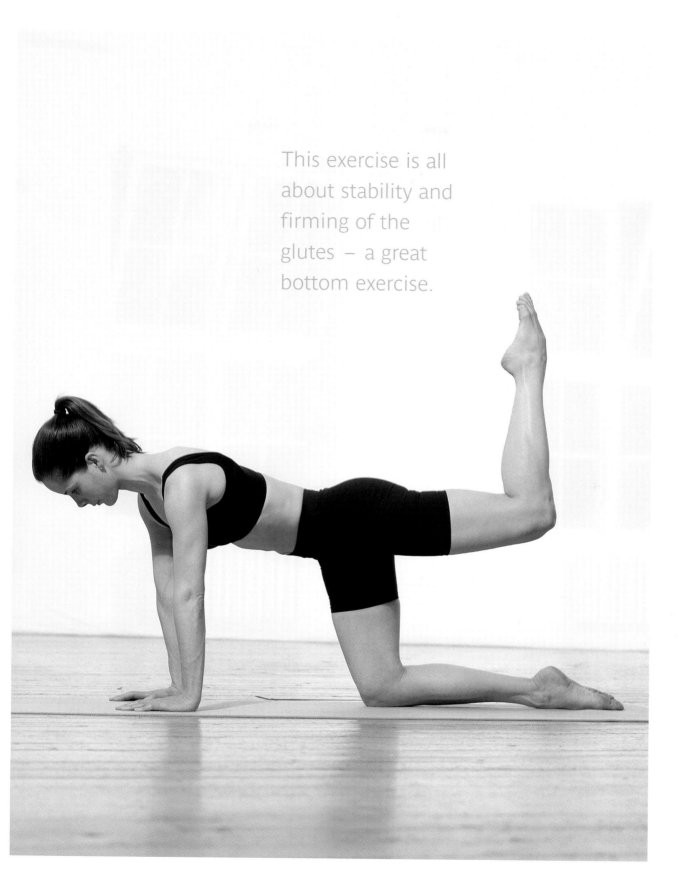

This exercise is all about stability and firming of the glutes – a great bottom exercise.

This exercise helps build strong
stomach muscles as you have to
support your alignment and
posture with your core/centre
the whole time.

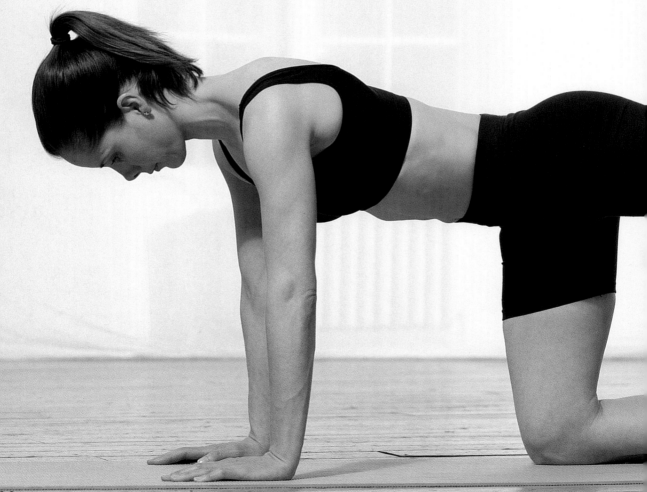

donkey

1 Get on to all fours on the floor. Knees should be under hips, arms under shoulders and head aligned with your back in a straight line, with stomach pulled in and shoulders pulled down.

2 Breathing normally, slide one leg along the floor and extend it into a lift, so it becomes an extension of your back (i.e. it's in line with your back). Hold for five counts and return to the starting position.

Repeat five times on one leg, then five times with the other.

TIP

ENSURE THAT YOU DON'T ROCK OR TRANSFER YOUR WEIGHT AS YOU LIFT YOUR LEG. HOLD IN YOUR CORE TO ENSURE STABILITY.

opposite arm and leg

1   Get onto all fours on the floor.
    Knees should be under hips,
    arms under shoulders and head
    aligned with your back in a
    straight line, with stomach
    pulled in and shoulders pulled
    down.

2   Inhale and, pulling in your
    abdominals to support your
    straight back, stretch out one
    arm and your opposing leg at
    the same time so both are in
    line with your body. Reach
    through your toes and fingers.

3   Exhale and return to the
    starting position and repeat
    with the other arm and leg.

Repeat five times on each leg,
alternating between them.

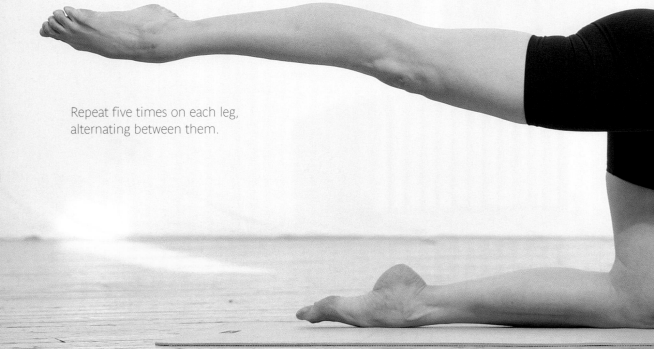

This exercise really works
your stomach muscles,
because you need to pull
them in to ensure stability.

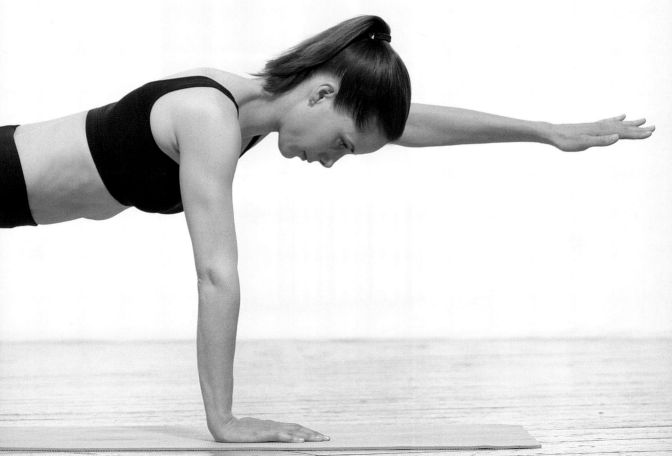

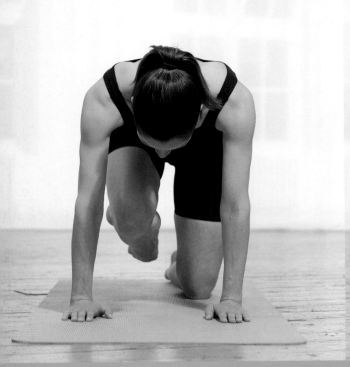 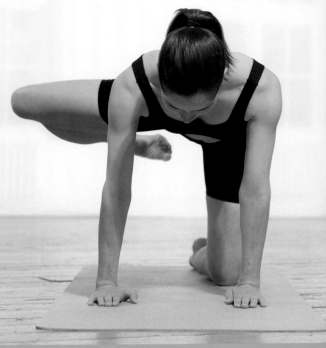

Although difficult, this exercise is good because it incorporates movement, stability and rotation.

hip circles

1 Get on to all fours on the floor. Knees should be under hips, arms under shoulders and head aligned with your back in a straight line, with stomach pulled in and shoulders pulled down.

2 Lift one knee towards your chest, then move it out to the side, then behind you, and finally return to the starting position. Keep your body still and stable. The key is to visualize making a large circle with your knee.

Repeat five times with one leg and then five times with the other.

> **TIP**
>
> MAKE SURE YOUR BELLY BUTTON IS PULLED IN TO YOUR SPINE AT ALL TIMES TO STABILIZE YOUR BACK AND STOP IT SINKING IN.

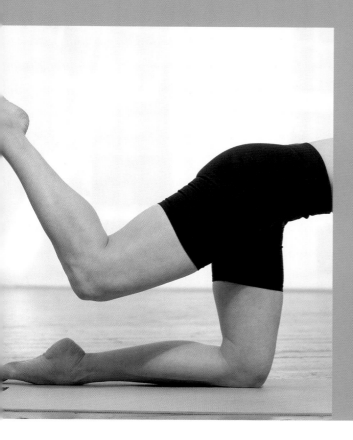

cat

1   Get on to all fours on the floor. Knees should be under hips, arms under shoulders and head aligned with your back in a straight line, with stomach pulled in and shoulders pulled down.

2   Inhale and, pulling your belly button to your spine, push upwards so that your upper body is curled (like a cat's back) and your bottom is taut. Relax your head and let it drop.

3   Exhale and move back into a straight back position, imagining your tailbone lengthening away at one end and your head at the other.

Repeat five times.

I could do these all day because they are a wonderful spine stretch and leave you feeling relaxed.

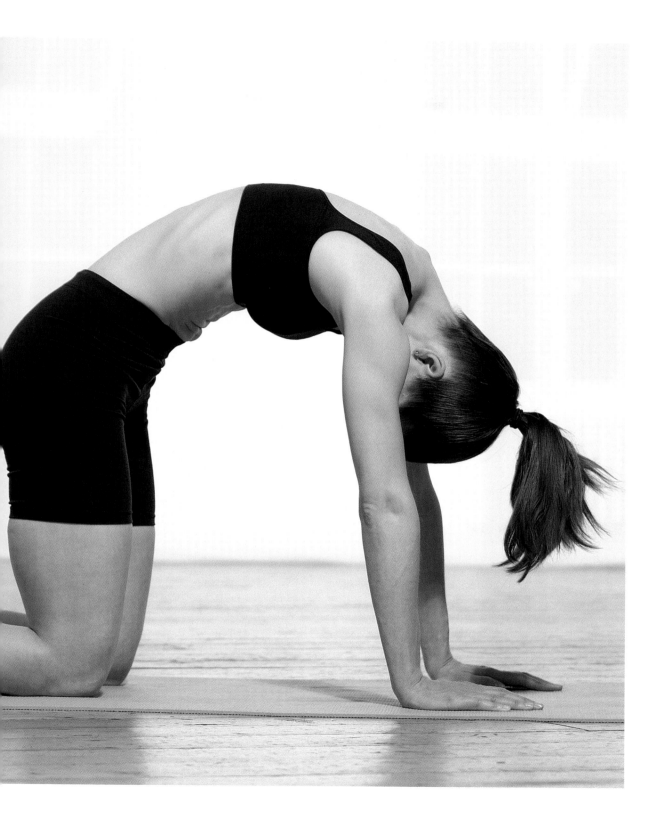

reverse cat

1   Get on to all fours on the floor.
    Knees should be under hips,
    arms under shoulders and head
    aligned with your back in a
    straight line, with stomach
    pulled in and shoulders pulled
    down.

2   Inhale, as you exhale imagine
    pushing your belly button
    down towards the floor (this
    should arch your back), and at
    the same time extend your
    breast bone out and forwards,
    keeping your shoulders down
    and your head aligned with
    your spine.

3   Move back into a straight back
    position.

    Repeat five times.

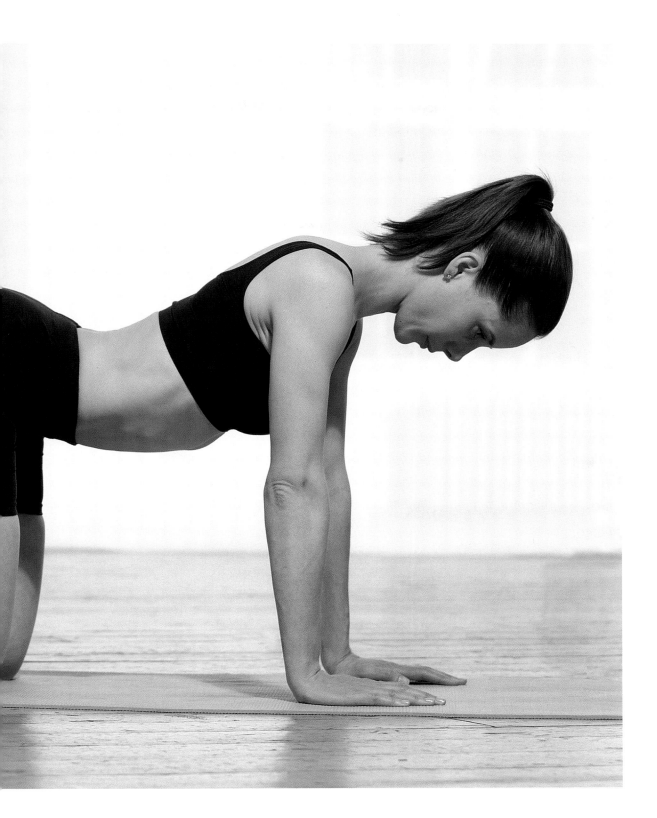

We are all guilty of tending to overwork one part of our body, especially if we want to tone up a specific area. Most women focus so much on the stomach that they forget about their lower back and sides. This area is very important because the muscles here can help give you upper-body length and a defined waist.

Most of us collapse into our waist as we stand and sit, and never think about lifting out of our sides so we have more length between our ribs and waist. Stretch out of your waist, and your spine will shoot upwards and your stomach will instantly get flatter.

The good news is that this area is easy to tone and stretch. The following exercises will help you pull out of your waist and give your body more length and strength. They will also help give you better posture and ensure you don't have shoulders up by your ears.

Remember, when you're lifting upwards your ribs should always stay dropped. There should never be a ledge above your waist; your ribs should be in a smooth line with your stomach.

prone

sphinx into a roll up

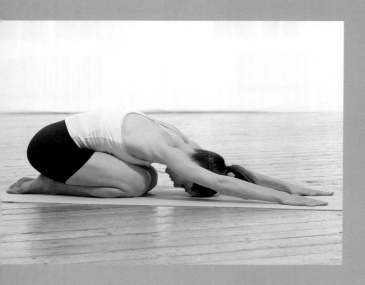

1 Face the ground on all fours and at the same time as drawing your bottom back (so that you are sitting back on your heels) extend your arms along the floor in front of you as far as they will go. Your forehead should now be on the floor. Keep your bottom on your heels.

2 From this prone position, inhale, draw your stomach up and slowly roll one vertebra at a time to come up to a kneeling position. Keep your bottom on your heels and let your arms drop to your sides.

3 Exhale and roll back down to the prone position.

Repeat five times.

TIP

FOR AN EXTRA STRETCH, WHEN LYING IN THE PRONE POSITION BREATHE DEEPLY INTO YOUR UPPER BACK TO STRETCH YOUR SPINE.

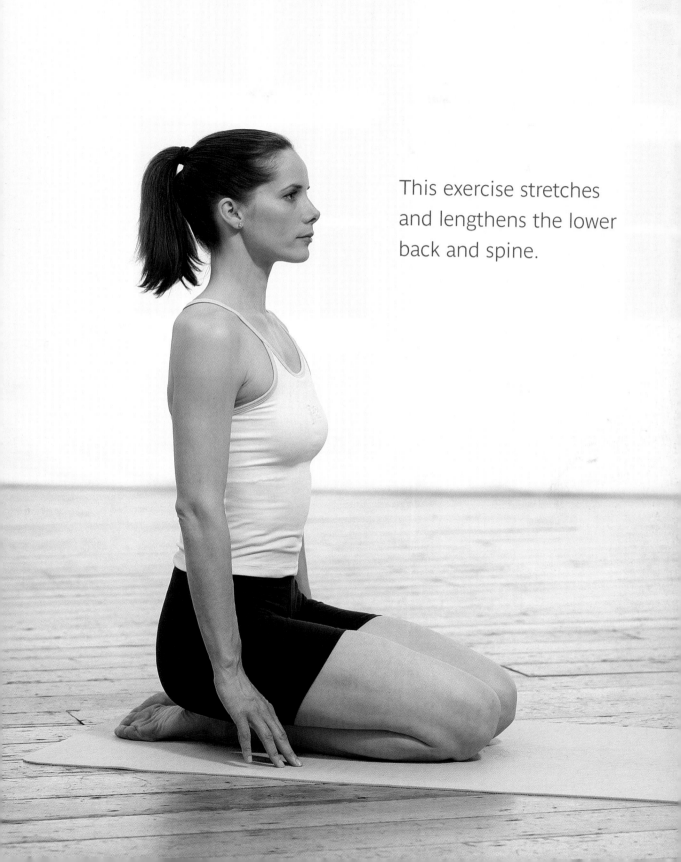

This exercise stretches
and lengthens the lower
back and spine.

glutes squeeze

1   Lie face down on the floor with
    a cushion under your forehead.
    Keep your arms by your sides
    with your palms face up and
    your stomach pulled in to
    support your lower back.

2   Inhale and squeeze your glutes
    (bottom muscles). Do not allow
    your hamstrings to contract;
    the movement should just
    come from your bottom. Hold
    for five counts.

3   Exhale and relax.

    Repeat ten times.

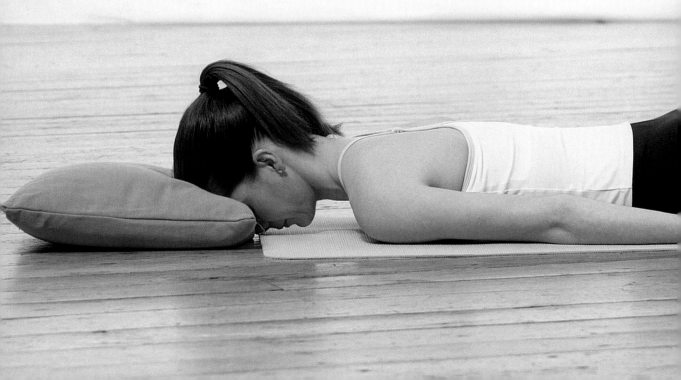

This exercise helps tone your bottom. Unlike many others, which work more than one set of muscles at the same time, this one specifically targets the glutes.

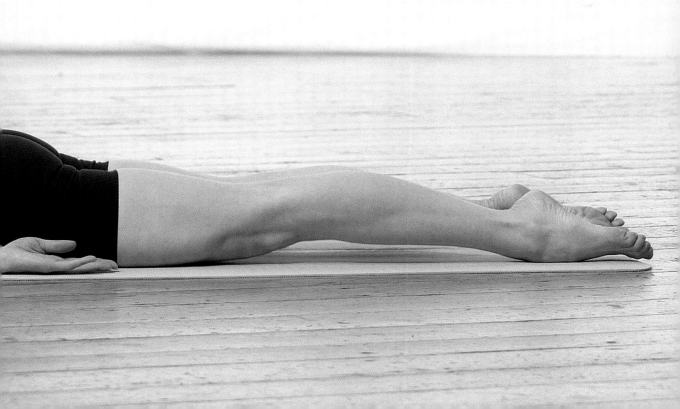

This is an easy, but very effective exercise.

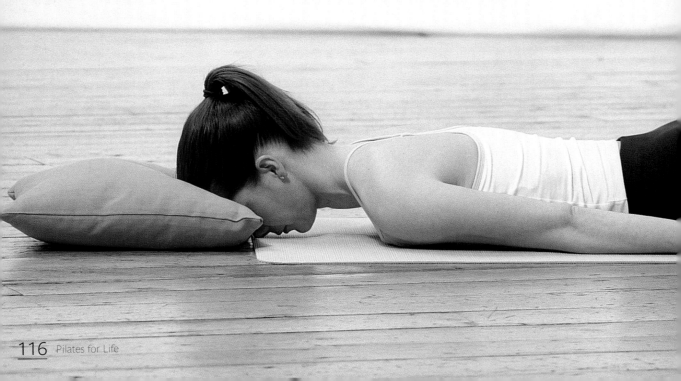

bent leg lift

1 Lie face down on the floor with a cushion under your forehead. Keep your arms by your sides, your palms face up.

2 Inhale, tighten your bottom muscles and lift one foot off the floor, bringing your leg up towards the ceiling so it is at a ninety-degree angle. Hold for two counts.

3 Exhale and return to the starting position.

Repeat five times on one leg and then five times on the other.

TIP

DON'T LET YOUR BACK ARCH. PULL IN YOUR STOMACH AND PELVIC FLOOR MUSCLES AND PUSH YOUR PUBIC BONE INTO THE FLOOR FOR EXTRA SUPPORT.

straight leg lift

1 Lie face down on the floor with
   a cushion under your forehead.
   Keep your arms by your sides,
   your palms face up.

2 Inhale, tighten your bottom
   muscles and lift one leg off the
   floor. Hold for four counts. Try
   not to let your leg waver.

3 Exhale and return to the
   starting position.

   Repeat five times on one leg
   and then five times on the
   other.

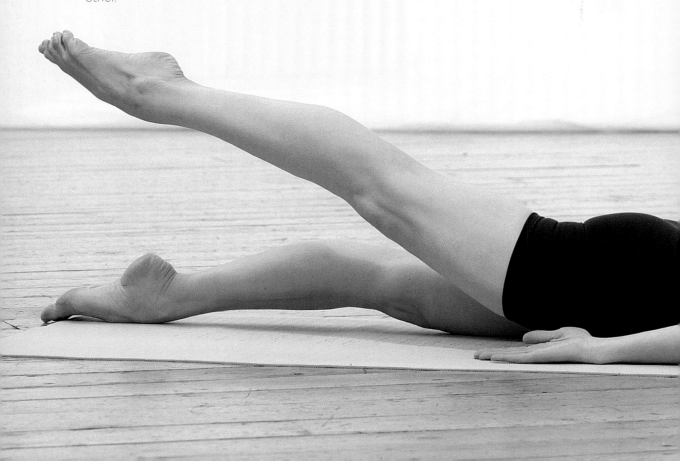

Works your inner thighs
and bottom because when
you're holding your leg off
the ground your inner thigh
and bottom muscles will
automatically engage.

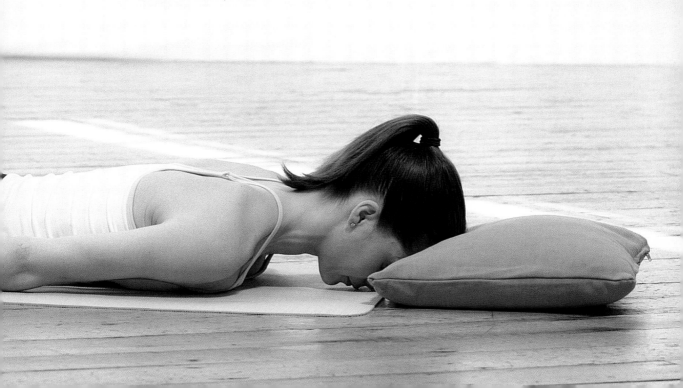

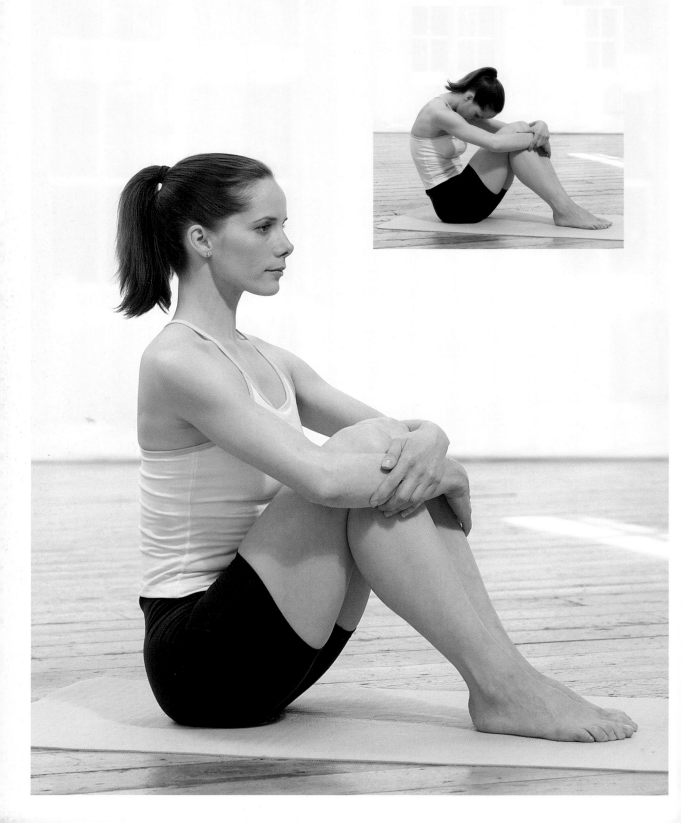

demetri abdominals

1 Sit on the floor with your back straight, your knees bent and your feet together. Wrap your arms around your knees.

2 Inhale and drop your chin towards your chest and form your body into a C-shape.

3 Pull your belly button in and push out your spine by imagining you're trying to reach a wall behind you with it.

4 Exhale and sit up, moving from the base of your spine upwards.

Repeat five times.

This is a nice extension for the spine, great for the stomach and a lovely stretch after being on all fours.

Balancing is all about good body alignment. If you do it right it's like a meditation because you need good concentration levels to focus your energy in order to stand and/or hold a position.

If you can balance well you know you're standing well. If you find you are wobbling, try fixing your eyes on a point to help you focus. Also, remember that to balance correctly you have to trigger your stomach muscles and engage your pelvic floor muscles. This is what helps your body maintain balance.

The other benefit in learning to balance is that in normal everyday life most of us are guilty of using the same muscles over and over. Repetitive movements such as always carrying a bag on the same shoulder or using one leg/side more than the other throws your body out of alignment. When this happens, your body starts to protect itself in strange ways. This is why it's important to counteract any bad habits you have developed by rebalancing and aligning your body with the following exercises.

balancing and lifting

clams (I)

1. Lie on one side with your knees bent in front of you, feet together (your soles should be in line with your back), and your stomach pulled in. Keep your lower arm extended under your head and your other hand on the floor in front of you for support.

2. Inhale and, making sure you don't sink into your waist, exhale and lift up your top knee so its pointing towards the ceiling, keeping your feet together and bottom taut (initiate the movement from your glutes). Make sure you keep your body aligned and don't physically turn your hip out.

3. Inhale and return to the starting position.

Repeat ten times on one leg, then turn over and repeat ten times on the other.

This is a very good bottom exercise.

> **TIP**
>
> WHEN DOING THIS EXERCISE, DON'T ROLL FORWARDS OR BACKWARDS ON YOUR HIPS. YOU SHOULD FEEL AS THOUGH YOU'RE LYING FLAT AGAINST A WALL WITH YOUR FEET, BACK AND HEAD TOUCHING IT.

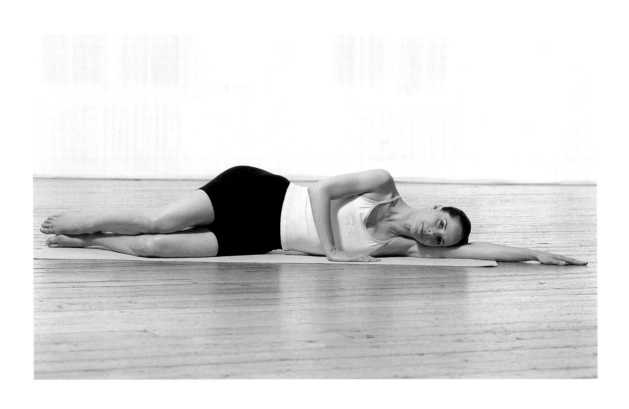

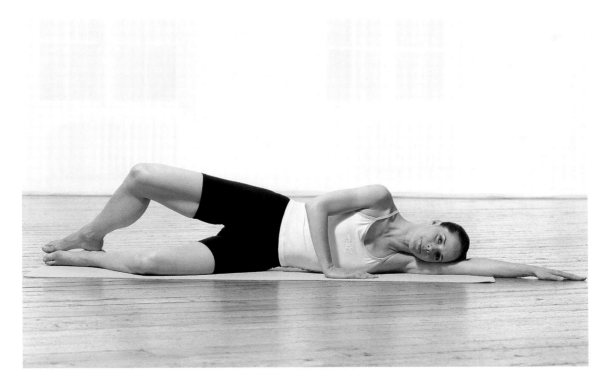

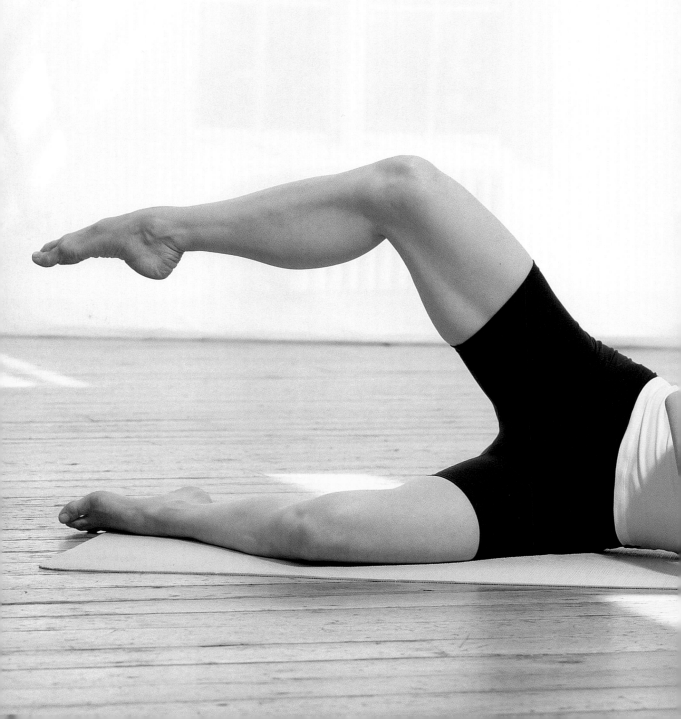

clams (II)

1 Lie on one side, with your knees bent in front of you, feet together (your soles should be in line with your back) and your stomach pulled in. Keep your lower arm extended under your head and place your other hand on the floor in front of you for support.

2 Inhale and, making sure you don't sink into your waist, lift up your top knee so it's pointing towards the ceiling. Keeping your leg in this position, lift it towards your hip. Exhale and lower your leg until your feet are touching.

Repeat ten times on one leg, then turn over and repeat ten times on the other.

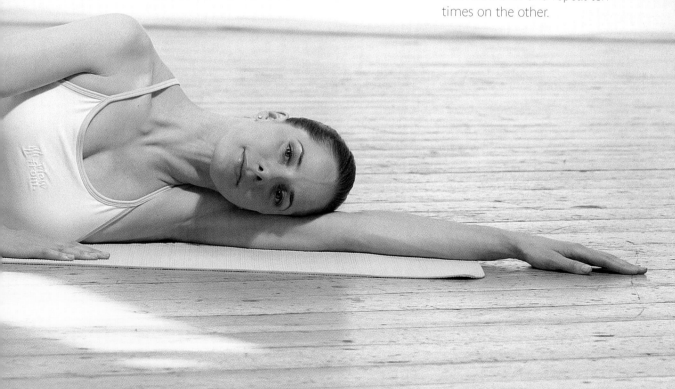

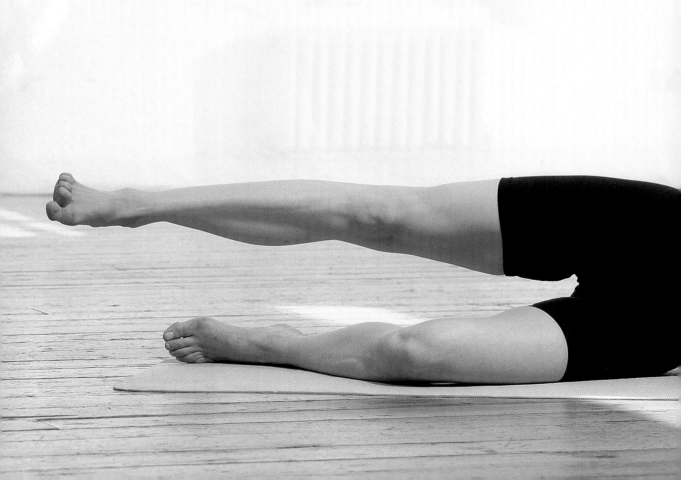

ronde de jambe

1   This means 'circle of the leg'.
    Lie on one side with your lower
    leg slightly bent and your top
    leg straight and aligned with
    your body. Keep your lower arm
    extended under your head and
    your other hand on the floor in
    front of you for support.

2   Breathing normally, lift your top
    leg slightly so it's in line with
    your top hip, and flex your foot.

3   In this position make small
    circles in one direction for four
    counts.

4   Return to the starting position
    then lift again and move your
    leg in the reverse direction for
    four counts.

    Repeat five times in each
    direction, then turn over and
    repeat on the other leg.

This exercise tones and firms
the inner and outer thighs.

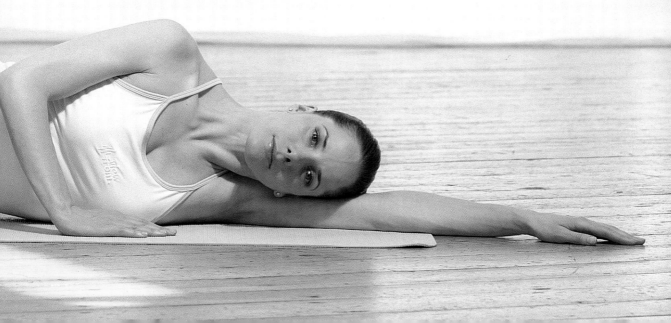

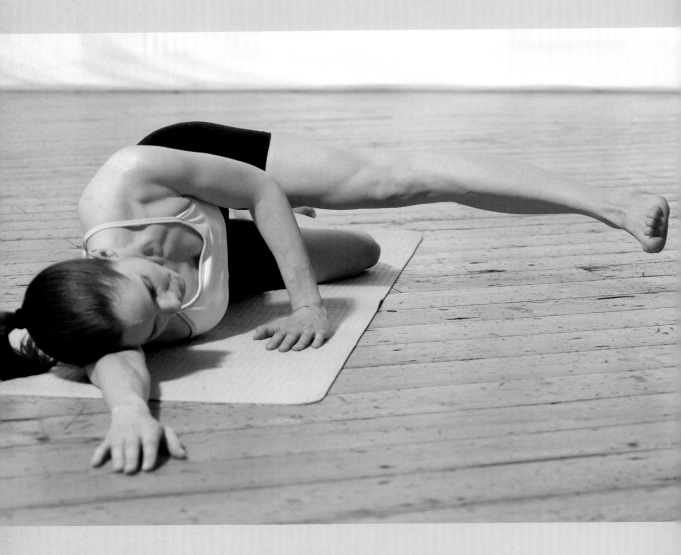

scissors

Very good for your legs
and stomach as it's all
about stability.

1   Lie on one side with your lower
    leg slightly bent and your foot
    flexed. Lift your top leg and
    carry it forward until it's
    perpendicular to the body. Keep
    your lower arm extended under
    your head and your other hand
    on the floor in front of you for
    extra support.

2   Breathing normally, lift your top
    leg so it's parallel to the floor.
    Tighten the buttock and,
    maintaining a continuous
    rotation in the hips, slowly
    move the leg back into line
    with the body and then
    forwards again.

    Repeat five times on one leg,
    then turn over and repeat five
    times on the other.

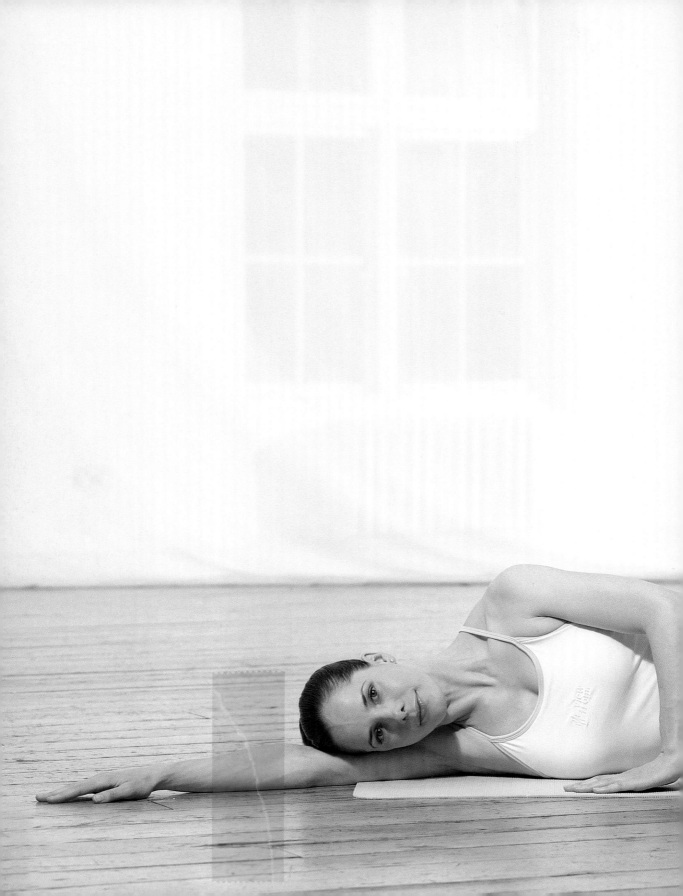

double leg lift

1   Lie on one side with both your
    legs straight and slightly in
    front of your body so you can
    see your feet. Keep your lower
    arm extended under your head
    and your other hand on the
    floor in front of you for
    support. Pull in your stomach
    muscles to support your back.

2   Breathing normally, extend
    both legs through the heel
    until they lift away from the
    floor. Hold for one count then
    return to the starting position.
    This whole movement should
    last four counts.

    Repeat five times on one side,
    then turn over and repeat five
    times on the other.

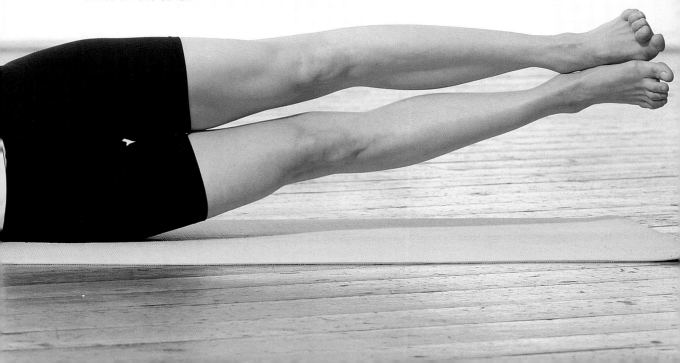

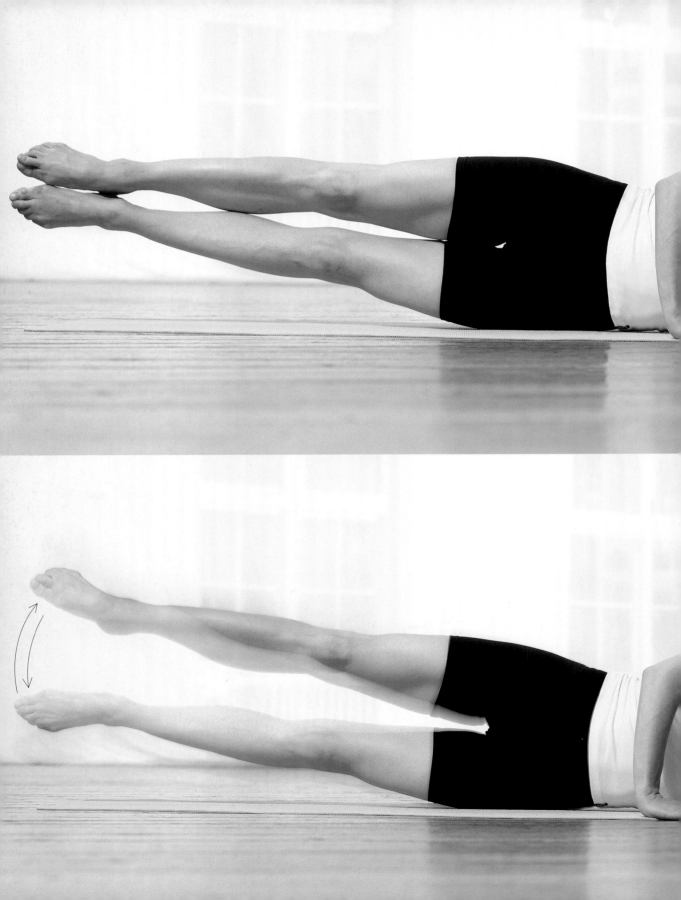

leg beats

1 Lie on one side with your legs straight and aligned with your body. Keep your lower arm extended under your head and your other hand on the floor in front of you for support.

2 Inhale and, pulling in your stomach muscles, lift both legs ten centimetres off the ground. Exhale.

3 Keeping both legs raised, inhale and pulse both legs in and out for ten beats, breathing normally. Bring both legs back to the floor.

Turn over and repeat on your other leg for ten beats.

Perfect for toning the inner thighs.

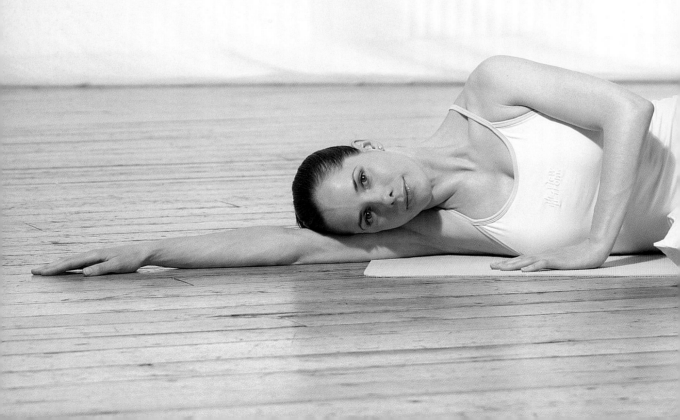

inside thigh lifts (I)

1   Lie on one side and put your
    upper leg and knee on a
    cushion in front of your body,
    keeping your bottom leg
    extended. Don't let your hip roll
    forward: it should remain level
    with your spine. Keep your
    lower arm extended under your
    head and your other hand on
    the floor in front of you for
    support.

2   Breathing normally, flex the
    foot and lift and lengthen the
    lower leg, extending your heel
    away from the floor. Hold for
    ten counts.

    Turn over and repeat on your
    other leg for ten counts.

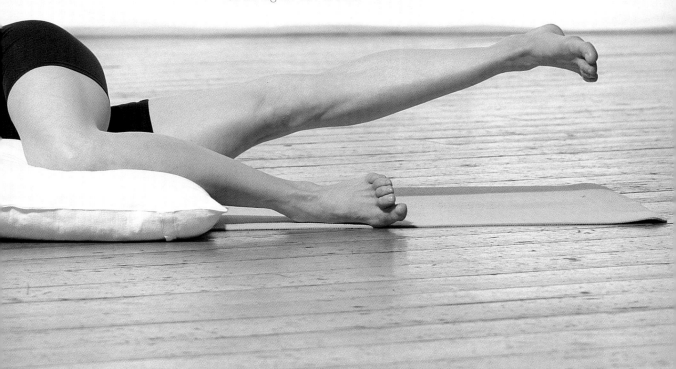

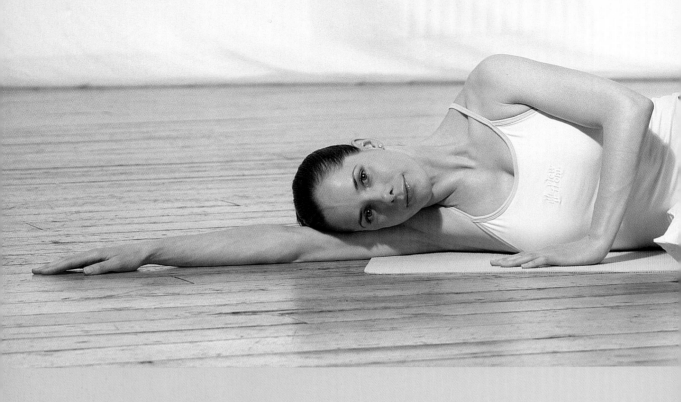

inside thigh lifts (II)

1   Lie on one side and put your
    upper knee on a cushion in front
    of your body, keeping your bottom
    leg extended. Don't let your hip
    roll forward: it should remain level
    with your spine. Keep your lower
    arm extended under your head
    and your other hand on the floor
    in front of you for support.

2   Breathing normally, flex the foot
    and lift and lengthen the lower
    leg, extending your heel away from
    the floor. Make five small circles
    with your leg in one direction,
    then five in the other direction.

    Turn over and repeat on your
    other leg.

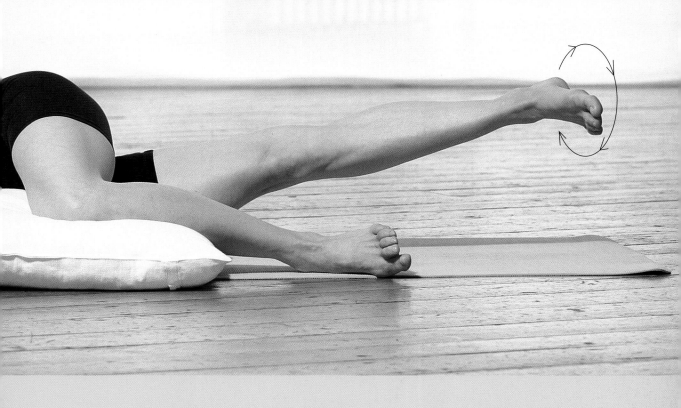

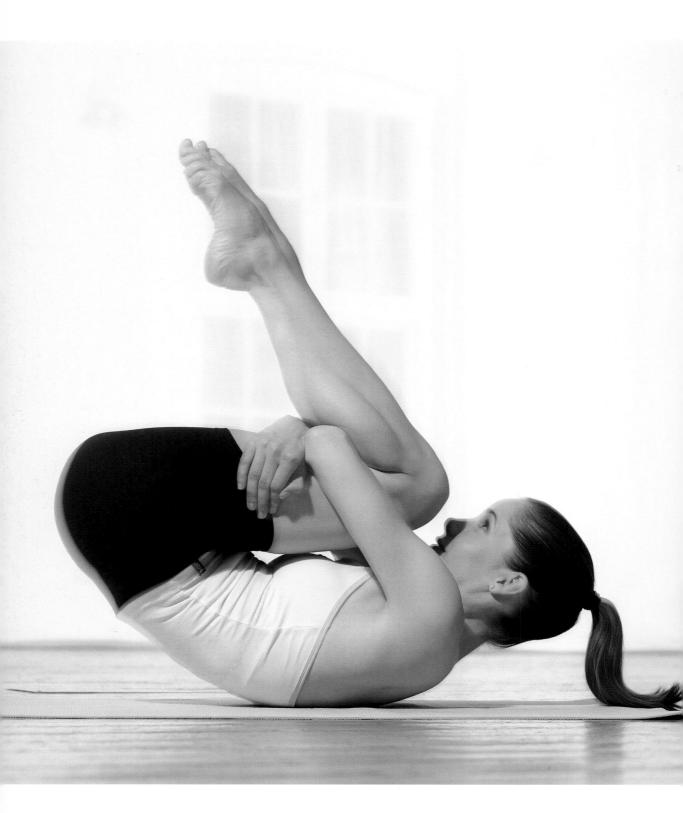

roll like a ball

This exercise is a wonderful spine massage.

1 You must use a mat for this exercise. Sit near the end of your mat with your knees bent and your feet together. Wrap your arms round your thighs and lift your feet off the mat, balancing on your tailbone. Tuck your chin into your chest (almost as though you have curled into a ball).

2 In this position inhale, pull your belly button in towards your spine, and roll backwards bringing your knees with you and keeping your head tucked in. Do not roll back on to your neck.

3 Exhale and, using your stomach to propel/rock you, roll forwards, then inhale and roll back again.

Repeat the rolling movement ten times without letting your feet touch the floor.

TIP

TO MAKE THIS EASIER, TRY HOLDING ON TO YOUR KNEES INSTEAD OF BEHIND YOUR THIGHS.

Arm work is also essential in Pilates because apart from firming up the upper arms and toning your biceps and triceps, these exercises help release tension in the neck, shoulders and upper back. They also stretch the chest muscles, which in turn help combat rounded shoulders and strengthen and open the chest area.

When you do the following exercises, remember to drop your shoulders consciously as you work, keep your ribs dropped and don't arch your back as you move your arms behind you. More importantly, when you move your arms backwards, keep the space between your shoulder blades and stretch through your fingers to keep your arms lengthened.

Finally, when rotating your arm through a movement, remember the rotation comes from the shoulder joint and not the wrist. To find the turn out, place your left hand at the top of your right arm, and as you turn your right arm out imagine the top of your arm rotating out and around the side.

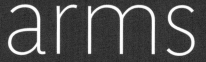
arms

hundreds for the upper arms

1. Stand square-on facing a mirror. Keep your legs hip-width apart and slightly bent, your shoulders pulled down and your stomach pulled in. Have your arms by your sides with palms facing backwards.

2. Keeping your arms straight, push them back as far as they will go. In this position beat your arms quickly back and forth in small movements for twenty counts. Aim to do a hundred beats while breathing normally.

TIP

THE AIM HERE IS TO IMAGINE YOU ARE IN WATER AND PUSHING YOUR ARMS BACK TO CREATE RESISTANCE.

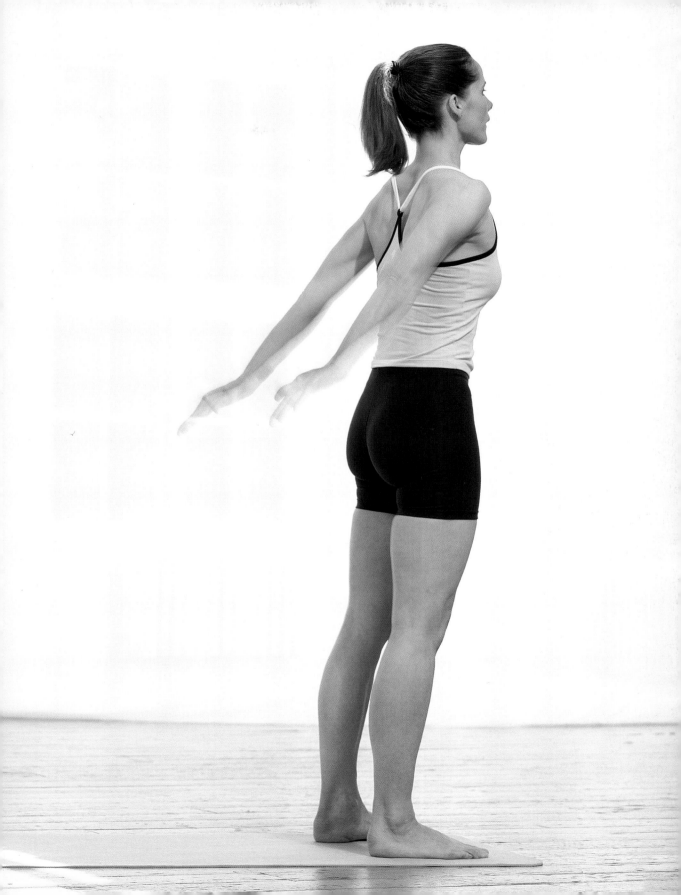

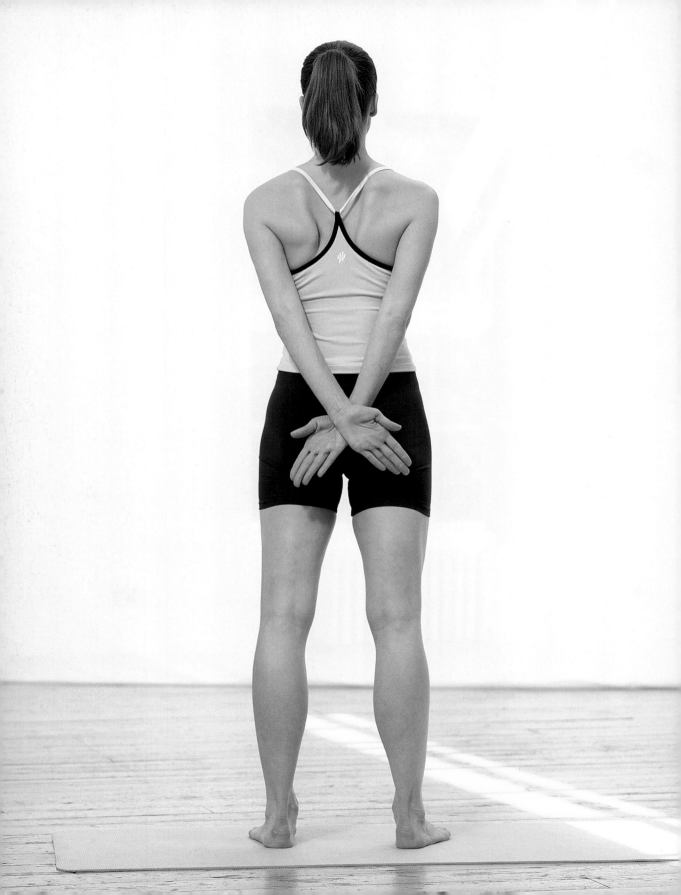

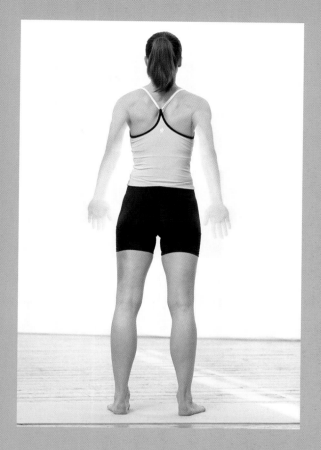

beating hundreds

1. Stand square-on facing a mirror. Keep your legs hip-width apart and slightly bent, your shoulders pulled down and your stomach pulled in. Have your arms by your sides with palms facing backwards.

2. Keeping your arms straight, push them back as far as they will go. Cross your arms behind you then swing them back out, then cross them behind you again. Continue this action in a controlled movement for twenty counts. As you cross palms behind you, you should alternate which one is on top; so left palm on top of right, swing arms back out, then right palm on top of left, and so on.

   Aim to do a hundred beats, breathing normally.

This and the previous exercise help to tone up the flabby parts of the upper arms that most women hate. I do these whenever I can.

waist twist

1 Stand square-on in front of a
   mirror with your feet hip-width
   apart and knees slightly bent.
   Imagine you are holding a
   football under each arm so that
   your arms are lifted and bent.
   Keep your stomach pulled in.

2 In this position let your arms
   feel heavy. Twist from your waist
   to one side, keeping your hips
   and head facing forwards. Let
   your arms swing to the front
   and back of your body in a
   perfect semi-circle.

3 Do a slow twist to each side
   and then three faster twists (as
   a guideline the two slow twists
   should take two counts and the
   three faster twists should also
   take two counts).

   Repeat ten times.

This exercise is brilliant for
the waist and stomach;
it will strengthen and slim
your waistline.

> **TIP**
>
> IMAGINE YOUR FINGERTIPS
> ARE FOLLOWING A HULA
> HOOP AROUND YOUR HIPS.

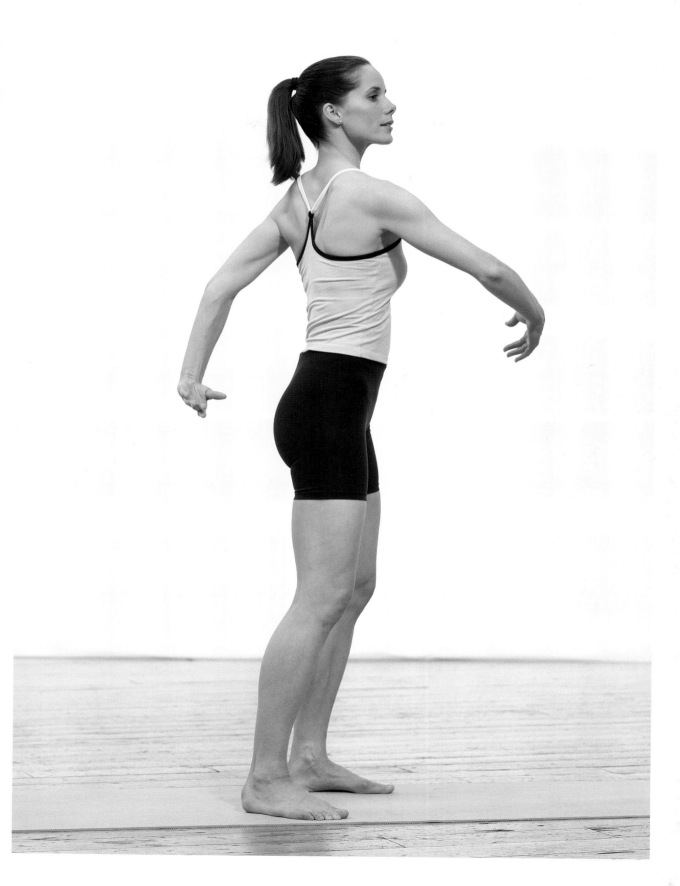

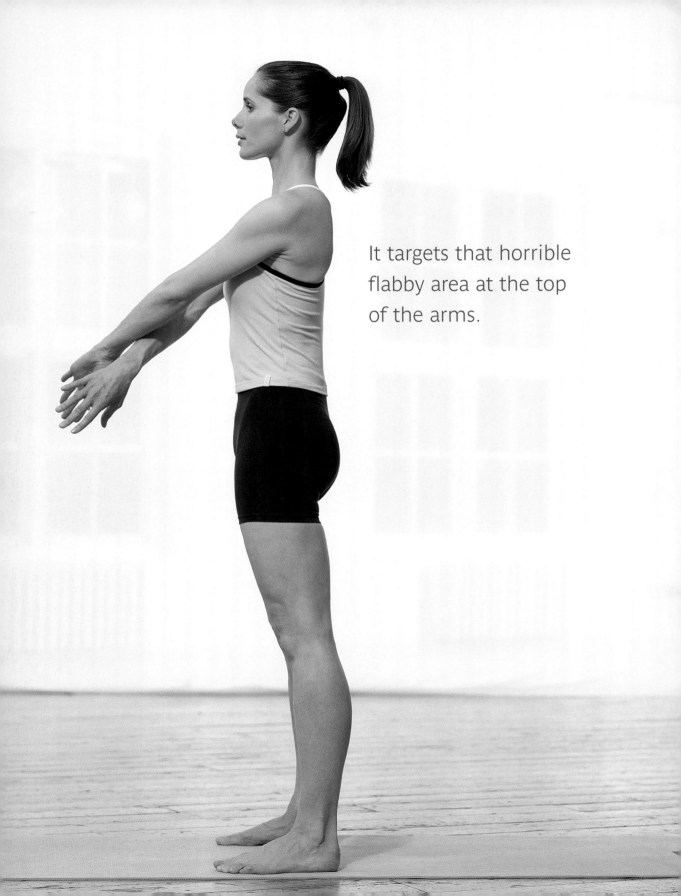

It targets that horrible flabby area at the top of the arms.

figures of eight

1 Stand square-on in front of a
mirror with your feet hip-width
apart and knees slightly bent,
arms by your sides and
stomach pulled in.

2 Inhale and, keeping your arms
straight, cross them in front of
you, palms facing each other
but not touching. Now turn
your arms out so that your
palms are facing up. Keeping
your shoulders down, swing
both arms outwards and behind
you as far as they will go.

3 Now turn your arms in so your
palms are facing backwards,
then swing them back to the
starting position.

4 Ensure the whole movement is
continuous and flowing. Both
arms should make one large,
curved figure of eight.

Repeat ten times.

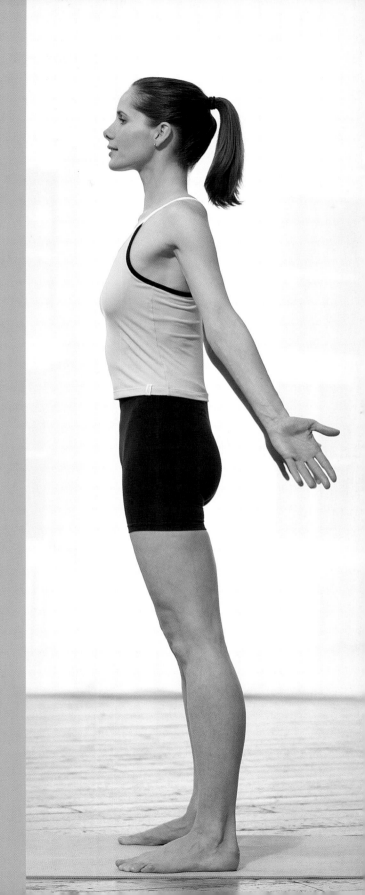

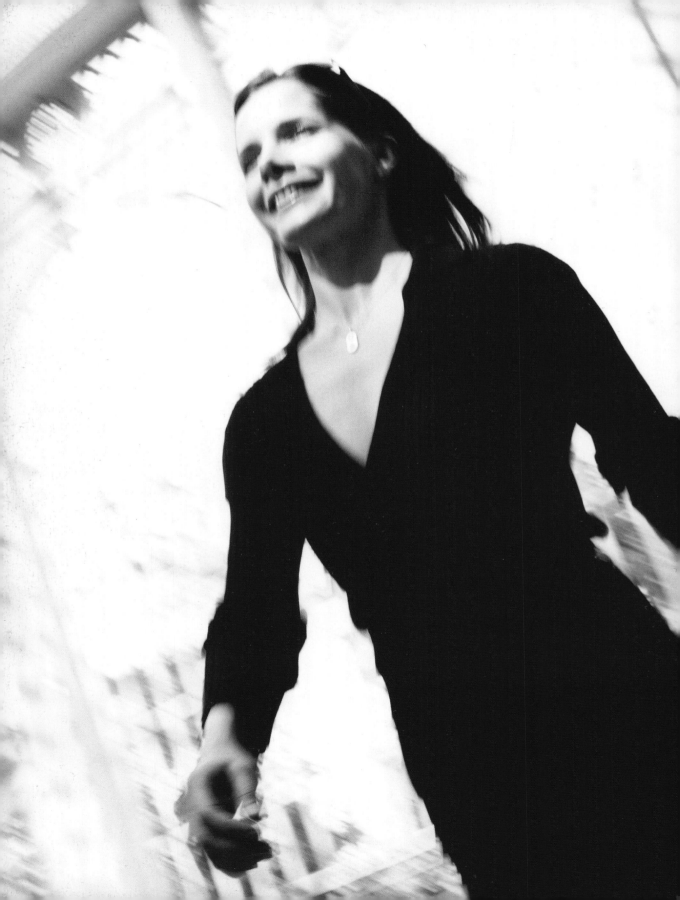

WARM DOWN

Stretching after exercise is essential because it helps your muscles to relax and reduces soreness and next-day stiffness (caused by a build up of lactic acid in the muscle). Try not to rush through the warm-down sequence, as each muscle needs to be held for at least thirty seconds to really stretch out.

side stretch

1 Stand up straight, with your feet hip-width apart and parallel, your stomach pulled in and ribs dropped (imagine them sliding down your front).

2 Inhale and allow one hand to slide down your side to your knee, letting go of your head at the same time. Hold for six counts.

3 Exhale and come back to centre.

Repeat five times then change sides.

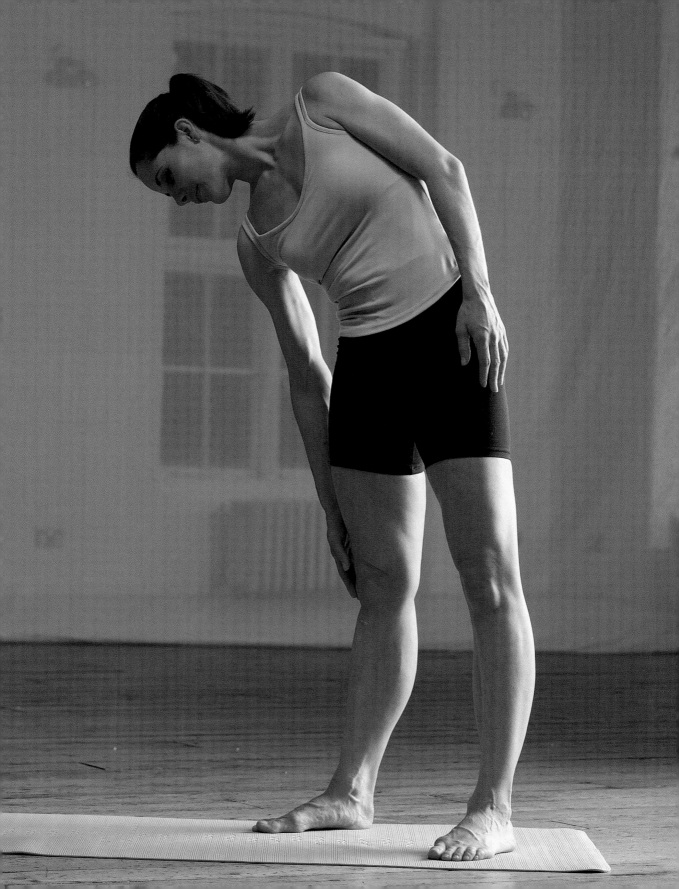

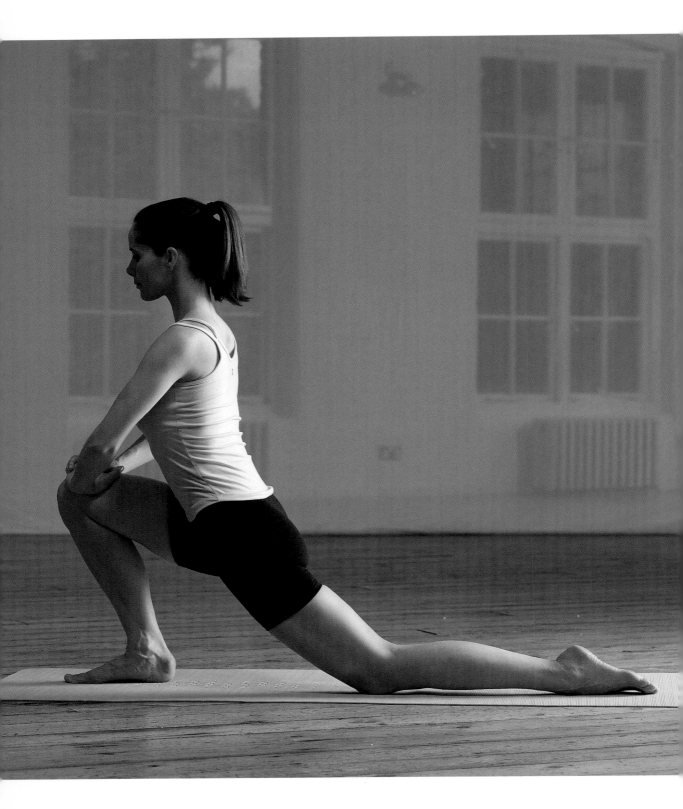

hip flexor

1   Kneel on both knees and then step forwards with your right foot so your leg is at a ninety-degree angle. Place both hands on your right knee.

2   Slide your left leg out behind you, keeping your knee on the floor, until you feel a stretch at the front of your left hip (this is your hip flexor).

3   Hold for thirty seconds then change legs.

4   To progress, push your hips forward and straighten your body, keeping your hands on your knee. In this position hold for thirty seconds, making sure your knee doesn't travel over your ankle.

Do one stretch on each leg.

quads

1 Stand up straight and place
your right hand against a wall
or chair for support. Keep your
feet parallel and hip-width apart
and your stomach pulled in.

2 Bend your left leg and, holding
your foot with your free hand,
pull it towards your bottom,
keeping your knees together,
back straight and hips aligned.
Hold for thirty seconds and
swap legs.

Do one stretch on each leg.

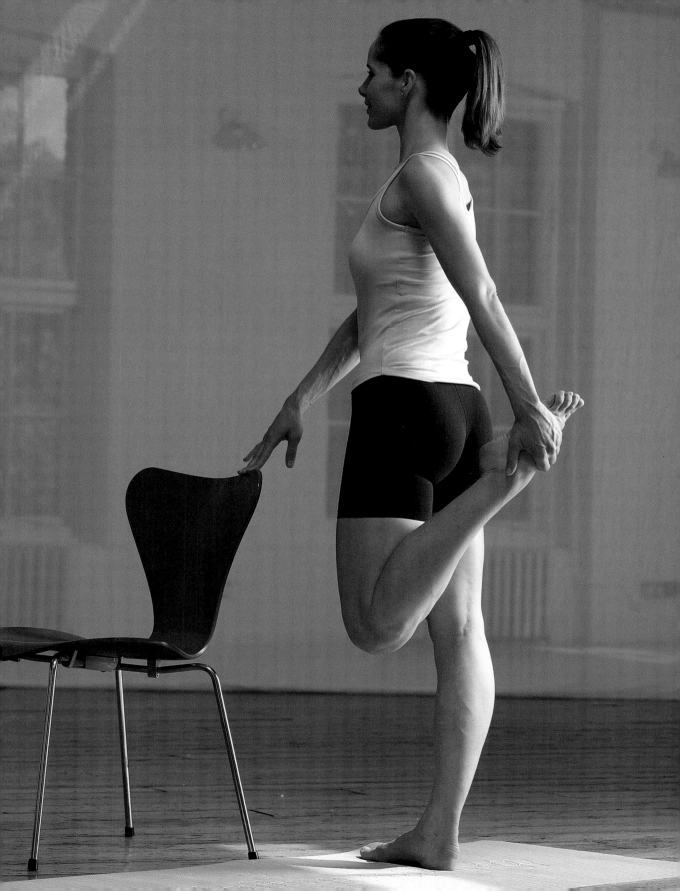

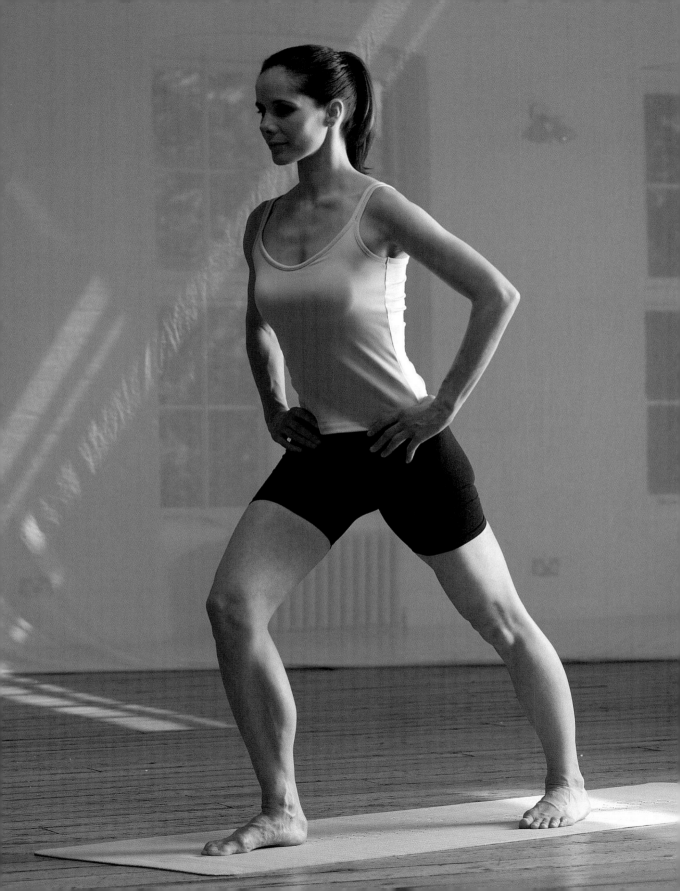

calf stretch

1. Stand with your feet together and then step back with one foot, bending the front leg slightly. Keep your back straight.

2. Push through the heel of your extended leg and tilt your body forward slightly (imagine there is a straight line running from your heel through the crown of your head).

3. Hold for thirty seconds and change legs.

Do one stretch on each leg.

TIP

IF YOU'RE A BEGINNER, USE A WALL FOR SUPPORT. STAND AN ARM'S LENGTH AWAY AND PLACE BOTH YOUR HANDS AT CHEST LEVEL ON THE WALL.

glute stretch

1 Lie on your back with your knees bent and place your right ankle across the left knee.

2 Lifting your head up clasp your hands around your left thigh. Inhale and pull your knee towards you (at the same time return your head to the floor).

3 Exhale and slowly pull your knee towards your chest. You should feel a stretch across your glutes (bottom). Hold for thirty seconds and release.

Repeat four times on one leg and then four times on the other.

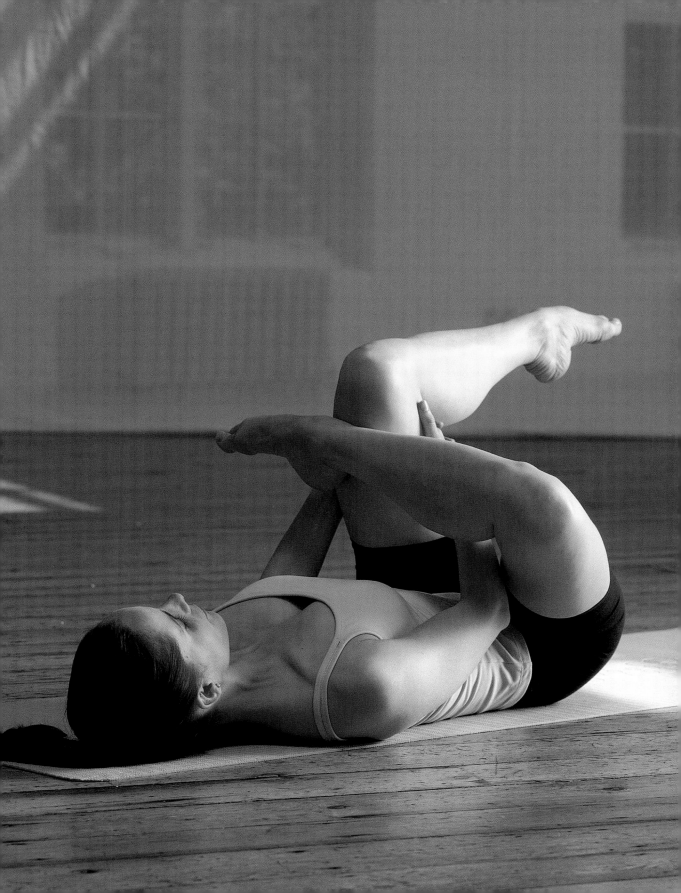

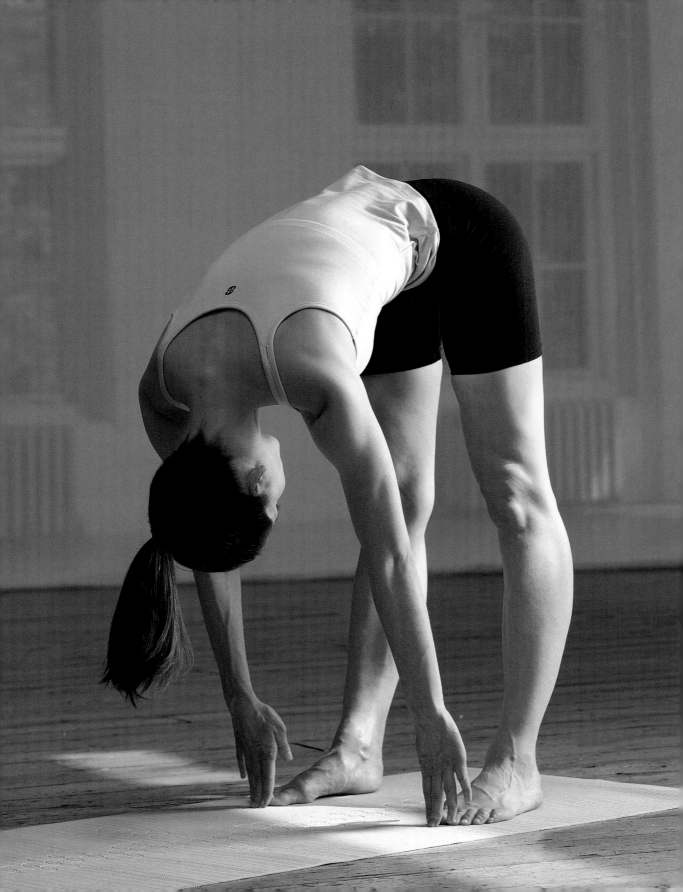

roll down

1 Stand with your feet hip-width apart and parallel, your belly button pulled in to your spine, your ribs dropped, your shoulders stable and your head in alignment with your spine.

2 Inhale and drop your head to your chest. Exhale and allow your arms to fall forwards as you roll down vertebra by vertebra. Keep your legs straight and, making sure you don't rock forwards or backwards as you roll, let go of your head and allow your hands to come as close to the floor as possible.

3 At the bottom hold for two counts, inhale and use your stomach muscles to curl upwards to the starting position.

Repeat three times.

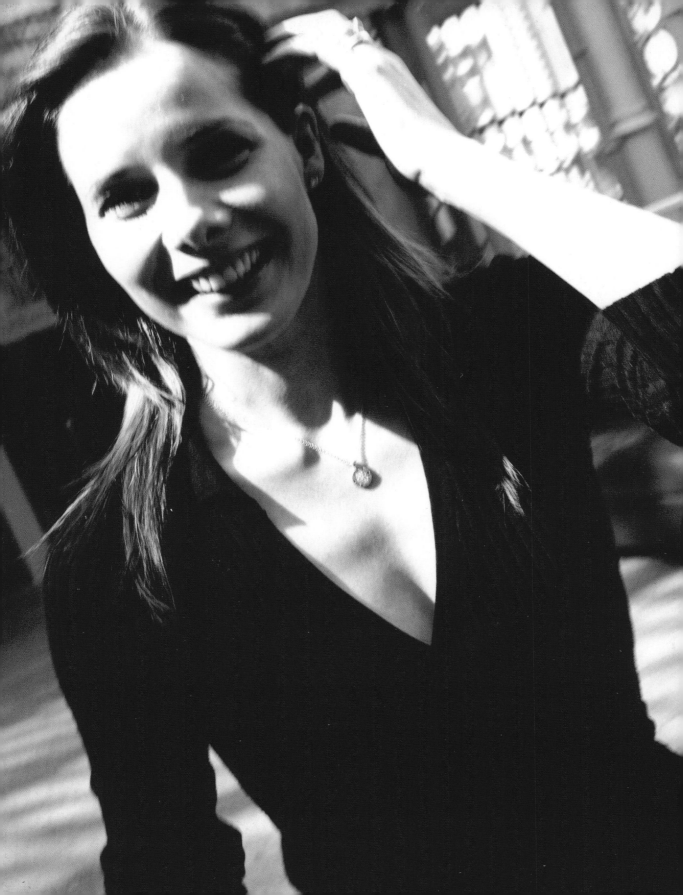

MINI
PROGRAMME

Once you have been through the whole Pilates plan a number of times, you can try my favourite mini programme. It takes just a few minutes a day to do, so is perfect if you are time starved, and it provides your entire body with a complete Pilates workout.

pelvic floor muscles – works your stomach and pelvic floor

single leg raise – works your hamstrings and glutes

double leg raise – works your hamstrings and glutes

obliques (modified) – works your waist and stomach muscles

dog – works your stomach

opposite arm and leg – works your stomach and aids stability

sphinx into a roll up – stretches your spine and works your stomach

clams (I) – works your inner thighs

inside thigh lifts (I) – works your inner thighs and bottom

figures of eight – tones your arms

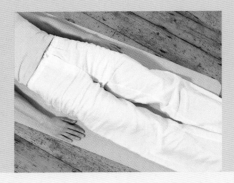

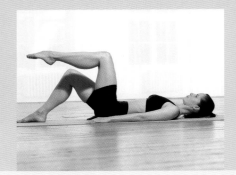

pelvic floor muscles

1   Lie down on the floor on your back with your legs straight and hip-width apart. Place your arms by your sides. Now, imagine peeing and then stopping mid flow – the muscles you are using are your pelvic floor muscles.

2   Squeeze these muscles together. This should allow you to feel your pelvic floor pull upwards to your stomach. Hold it for four counts, then relax.

Repeat ten times.

single leg raise

1   Lie on the floor with your knees bent at a ninety-degree angle, feet parallel and hip-width apart, your belly button pulled towards your spine and your arms by your sides.

2   Slowly inhale and at the same time pull your stomach muscles in and let one leg float up off the floor bringing the knee over the hip, keeping your leg at a ninety-degree angle. Hold for two counts, and on the exhale return your leg to the floor in two counts.

Repeat ten times on each leg, alternating between them.

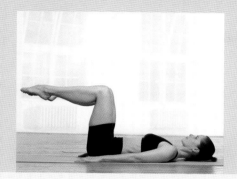

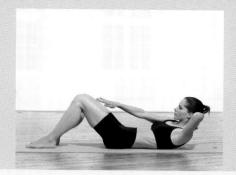

double leg raise

obliques (modified)

1 Lie on the floor with your knees bent at a ninety-degree angle, feet parallel and hip-width apart, your belly button pulled towards your spine and your arms by your sides.

2 Slowly pull your stomach muscles in, breathing normally, then let one leg float up until the knee is over the hip, keeping your leg at a ninety-degree angle. Then bring your other leg up to the same position and hold for two counts. Allow the first leg to go back down in two counts and then the other. Control both your legs on the way down to the floor with your stomach muscles; don't push down with your hands.

Repeat ten times.

1 Lie on the floor with your knees bent at a ninety-degree angle, feet parallel and hip-width apart. Place one hand behind your head and the other by your side. Inhale.

2 As you exhale, scoop in your abdominals and curl your head and chest off the floor (fix your gaze on your knees), and twist as you move your free arm towards your opposing knee.

3 Exhale and slowly curl back down to the floor and repeat with your other arm.

Repeat five times on each side, alternating between them.

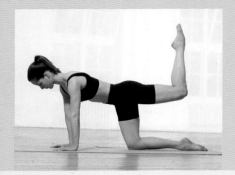

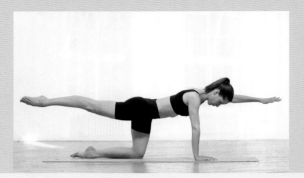

dog

1   Get onto all fours on the floor.
    Knees should be under hips,
    arms under shoulders and head
    aligned with your back in a
    straight line, with your stomach
    pulled in and shoulders pulled
    down.

2   Breathing normally, lift one leg
    off the floor and, keeping it
    bent at ninety degrees, extend
    your foot to the ceiling,
    bringing your knee in line with
    your hip. Then return it to the
    starting position.

    Repeat five times on each leg,
    alternating between them.

opposite arm and leg

1   Get onto all fours on the floor.
    Knees should be under hips,
    arms under shoulders and head
    aligned with your back in a
    straight line, with stomach
    pulled in and shoulders pulled
    down.

2   Inhale and, pulling in your
    abdominals to support your
    straight back, stretch out one
    arm and your opposing leg at
    the same time so both are in
    line with your body. Reach
    through your toes and fingers.

3   Exhale and return to the
    starting position and repeat
    with the other arm and leg.

    Repeat five times on each leg,
    alternating between them.

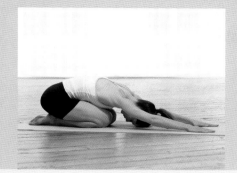

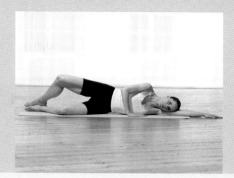

sphinx into a roll up

clams (i)

1 Face the ground on all fours and at the same time as drawing your bottom back (so that you are sitting back on your heels) extend your arms along the floor in front of you as far as they will go. Your forehead should now be on the floor. Keep your bottom on your heels.

2 From this prone position, inhale, draw your stomach up and slowly roll one vertebra at a time to come up to a kneeling position. Keep your bottom on your heels and let your arms drop to your sides.

3 Exhale and stretch back down to the prone position.

Repeat five times.

1 Lie on one side with your knees bent in front of you, feet together (your soles should be in line with your back), and your stomach pulled in. Keep your lower arm extended under your head and your other hand on the floor in front of you for support.

2 Inhale and, making sure you don't sink into your waist, exhale and lift up your top knee so its pointing towards the ceiling, keeping your feet together and bottom taut (initiate the movement from your glutes). Make sure you keep your body aligned and don't physically turn your hip out.

3 Inhale and return to the starting position.

Repeat ten times on one leg, then turn over and repeat ten times on the other.

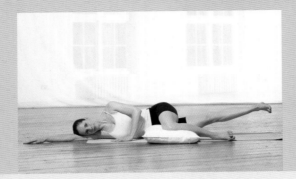
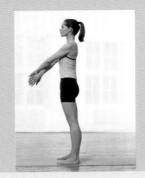

inside thigh lifts (I)

1 Lie on one side and put your upper leg and knee on a cushion in front of your body, keeping your bottom leg extended. Don't let your hip roll forward: it should remain level with your spine. Keep your lower arm extended under your head and your other hand on the floor in front of you for support.

2 Breathing normally, flex the foot and lift and lengthen the lower leg, extending your heel away from the floor. Hold for ten counts.

Turn over and repeat on your other leg for ten counts.

figures of eight

1 Stand square-on in front of a mirror with your feet hip-width apart and knees slightly bent, arms by your sides and stomach pulled in.

2 Inhale and, keeping your arms straight, cross them in front of you, palms facing each other but not touching. Now turn your arms out so that your palms are facing up. Keeping your shoulders down, swing both arms outwards and behind you as far as they will go.

3 Now turn your arms in so your palms are facing backwards, then swing them back to the starting position.

4 Ensure the whole movement is continuous and flowing. Both arms should make one large, curved figure of eight.

Repeat ten times.

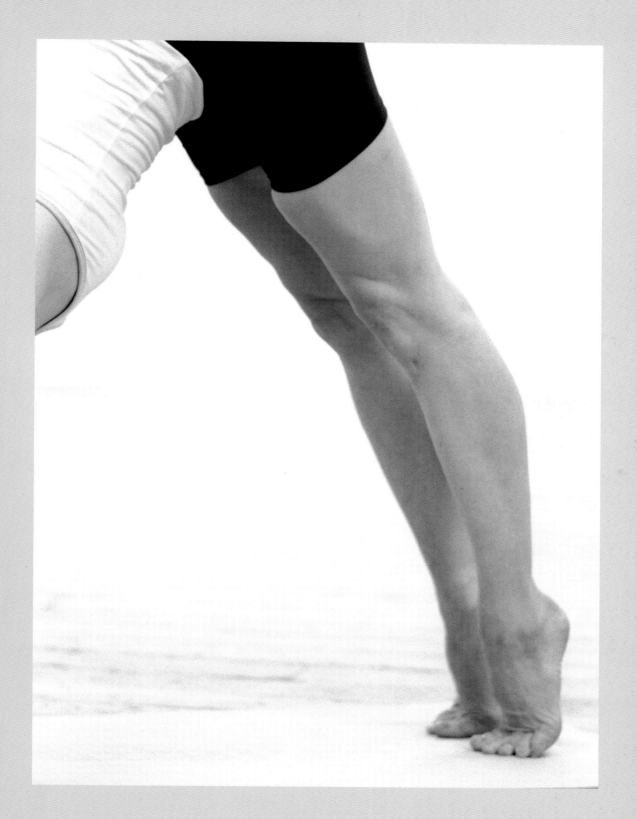

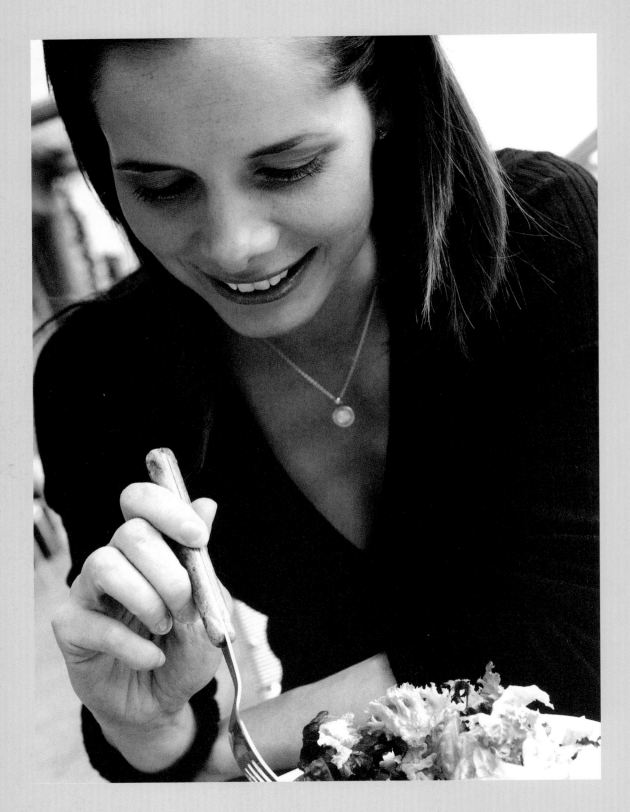

Conclusion

Healthy living is about more than exercise: it's also about looking after yourself, eating well and taking time out from a busy schedule to relax and enjoy your life. To reap the best benefits from Pilates I suggest the following to help boost your energy and maximize the effects of this programme.

- Drink more water. Water is the best energy boost you can give yourself so aim to drink at least 1.5 litres a day. Keep sipping it continuously whilst doing the programme, and don't drink it cold – it's best at room temperature.

- Avoid mindless snacking on foods with little nutritional value. Dried fruits such as apricots are good for energy, and nibbling on these will get you through the day.

- Also eat plenty of fruit to boost your immune system, and for a flat stomach limit your wheat intake (bread and pasta).

- Finally, for a healthy body that's without aches and pains, keep yourself as active as possible in any way you can throughout the day.

Glossary

A COUNT

This is the time it takes you to make one breath (an inhale and exhale).

ALIGNMENT

During every Pilates exercise the body should be in alignment. This means all the joints are in line and symmetrical to each other.

BICEPS

These are the muscles at the front of your upper arms, and the ones you use when you lift up objects.

CORE/CENTRE

Every movement in Pilates is initiated from the core. This is the band of muscles – the transversus abdominis, and the obliques – which wrap around your body like a corset helping to support you and give you good posture. Building strength here is essential for a healthy spine and flat stomach.

DRAWING IN OF THE CORE

This is the belly button to the spine movement, which engages your core muscles.

HAMSTRINGS

These are the muscles that run up the backs of your legs from your knees to your buttocks.

HIP FLEXORS

The hip flexors are the muscles of the hip area, which are used when you bring your knee to your chest or lift up the knee.

HYPERMOBILITY

This is a common condition in many people and occurs when there is too much movement in a joint. This can make the joint unstable and tends to cause the body to rock during movement. You may find your knees sway backwards slightly when straight. If this is what happens to you, keep your knees softly bent when standing in parallel.

GLUTES

These are the muscles in your buttocks that lie above your hamstrings.

LENGTHENING

A feeling rather than a forced movement, whereby you imagine your head slowly stretching away from your toes.

MOMENTUM

This is the force with which you exert your movements to get your body through a hard exercise. In Pilates, movement should not come from momentum, but from core strength to help build and tone muscle. The key is to control all movements and not rely on speed.

NEUTRAL SPINE

The position of your spine when you're lying on the floor. You should have a small natural curve to your lower back.

OBLIQUES

These are your side abdominal muscles, which lie around your waist.

POSTURE

This is the way you hold your body; not just when you're standing, but also when you are sitting and bending to lift objects.

QUADS

These are the front of the thigh muscles that run from your hip to your knee.

RONDE DE JAMBE

This means literally 'circle of the leg' – see the relevant exercise for more details.

SCOOPING

See *drawing in of the core*

SHOULDER STABILIZATION

The sliding of your shoulder blades down your back to ensure that your shoulders are in the right position for an exercise (i.e. not up around your ears).

SOFTENING

This is another way of saying be careful not to lock into your joints (see *hypermobility*) and keep your legs and arms lengthened but soft.

STABILIZATION

This is where you hold your bones in place and allow a movement to take place around the joint. For instance, keeping your hips stable (stationery) and allowing the leg to rotate around the hip joint.

TURN OUT

A rotation of the leg from the hip joint not the foot, or rotation of the arm from the shoulder not the wrist.

YOGA

Yoga is also a mind–body technique, but differs from Pilates in some ways, including the use of the breath during movements.

Darcey's story

Darcey Bussell was born in London on 27 April 1969. At the age of thirteen she was accepted into the Royal Ballet School where she studied for five years before joining Sadler's Wells Royal Ballet in 1987. In September 1989 Darcey joined the Royal Ballet, becoming a First Soloist; three months later she was promoted to Principal – she was just twenty years old. She has danced for the New York City Ballet and the Kirov Ballet of St Petersburg, and has guested internationally with several other companies.

Darcey was awarded Dancer of the Year in 1990 by *Dance & Dancers* magazine. That same year she also received both the Sir James Garreras Award for the most promising newcomer and the *Evening Standard* Ballet Award. She was joint winner of the *Cosmopolitan* Achievement Award in the Performing Art category in 1991 and was entitled an Officer of the Order of the British Empire (OBE) in the 1995 New Year's Honours List.

Darcey and her husband Angus have two daughters, Phoebe (born June 2001) and Zoe (born February 2004).

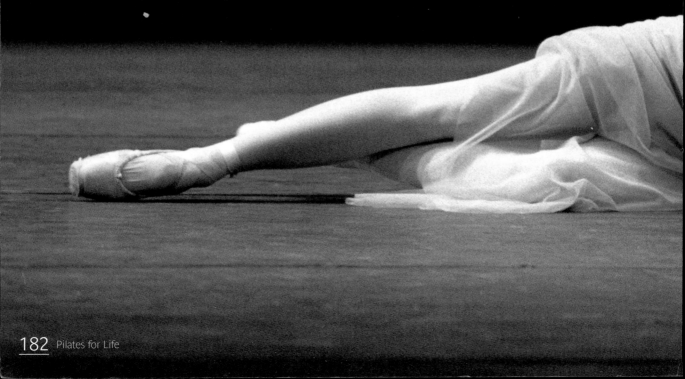

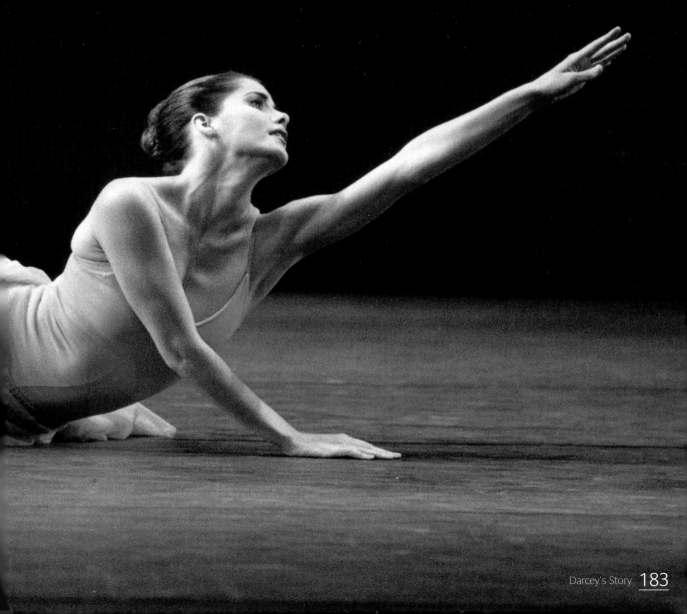

ROYAL BALLET SCHOOL
Concerto (principal role)

THE ROYAL BALLET
Kenneth MacMillan Productions
The Prince of the Pagodas (Princess Rose) – created
Winter Dreams (Masha) – created
Manon (title role)
Romeo and Juliet (title role)
Song of the Earth (leading role)
Elite Syncopations (leading role)
Requiem (Agnus Dei)
Mayerling (Mitzi Caspar)
Anastasia (Mathilde Kschessinska)

Classical Repertory
Swan Lake (Odette/Odile)
The Sleeping Beauty (Princess Aurora)
The Nutcracker (Sugar Plum Fairy)
La Bayadere (Nikiya and Gamzatti)
Giselle (title role)
Raymonda Act III (title role)

Balanchine Repertory
Rubies
Stravinsky: Violin Concerto (Aria I)
Agon (central role)
Symphony in C, Second Movement (central role)
Tchaikavsky – pas de deux
Apollo (Terpsichore)
Prodigal Son (Siren)
Duo Concertant (central role)
Ballet Imperial (central role)
Serenade – pas de deux

Frederick Ashton Productions

Cinderella

Monotones II

Les Illuminations (Sacred Love)

Birthday Offering, Beriosova Variation – *pas de deux*

Les Rendezvous – *pas de deux*

Created Leading Roles

Twyla Tharp's *Mr Worldly Wise* (Mistress Truth-on-Toe)

Matthew Hart's *Dances With Death*

Christopher Wheeldon's *Pavane Pour Une Infante Defunte* – *pas de deux*

Glen Tetley's *Amores sextet*

Mark Baldwin's *Towards Poetry*

John Neumeier's *Lento* – *pas de deux*

Christopher Wheeldon's *There Where She Loves*

Michael Corder's *Dance Variations* (principal role)

Christopher Wheeldon's *Tryst* (leading role)

Other Leading Roles

William Forsythe's *In the Middle, Somewhat Elevated*

William Forsythe's *Herman Scherman* – *pas de deux*

Glen Tetley's *La Ronde* (the Prostitute)

Ninette de Valois' *Checkmate* (the Black Queen)

Ashley Page's *…Now Languorous, Now Wild…* – *pas de deux*

Twyla Tharp's *Push Comes to Shove*

Jerome Robbin's *The Concert*

Antony Tudor's *Lilac Garden* (Caroline)

Stephen Baynes's *Beyond Bach* (the leading couple with Jonathon Cope)

Mark Morris' *Gong*

Natalia Makarov's *The Sleeping Beauty* (Aurora)

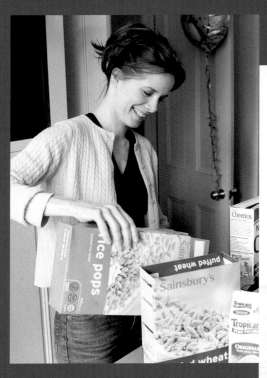

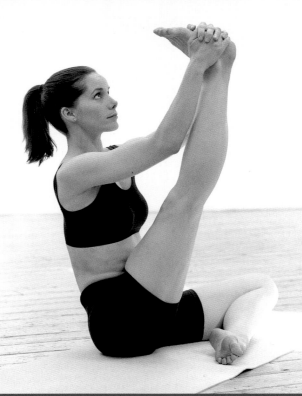

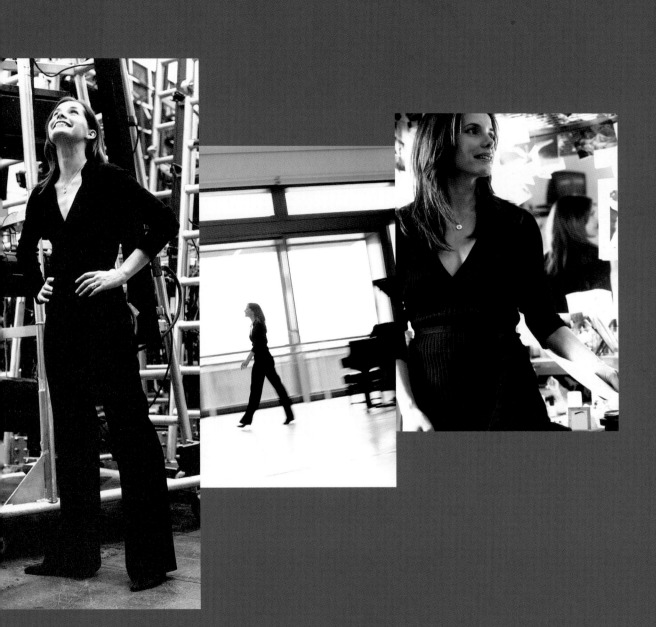

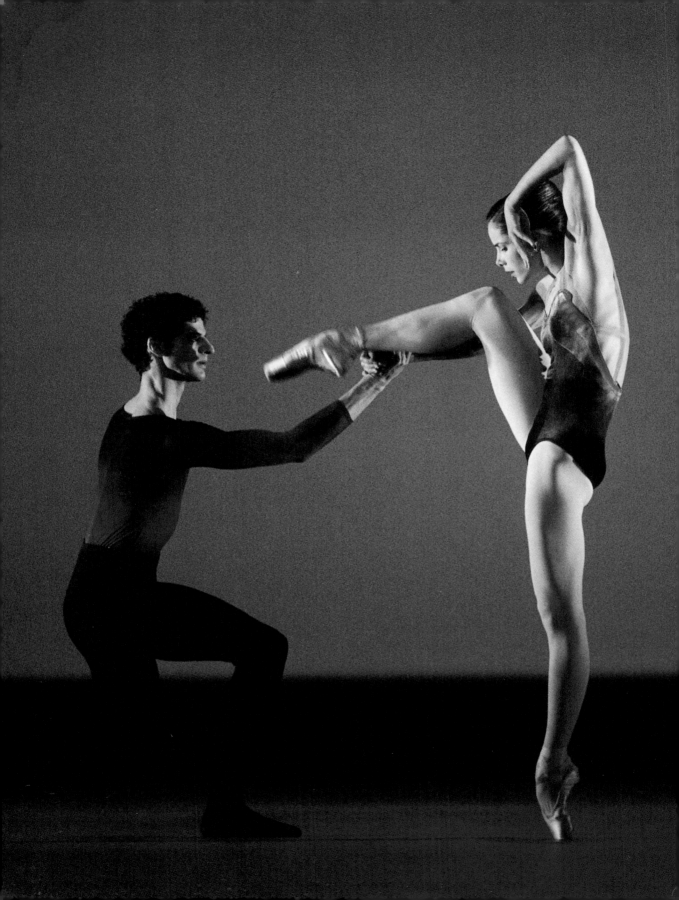